Dear So

LAUREN'S
VISION

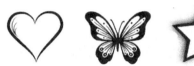

Lim H.P.H.

Lisa C.

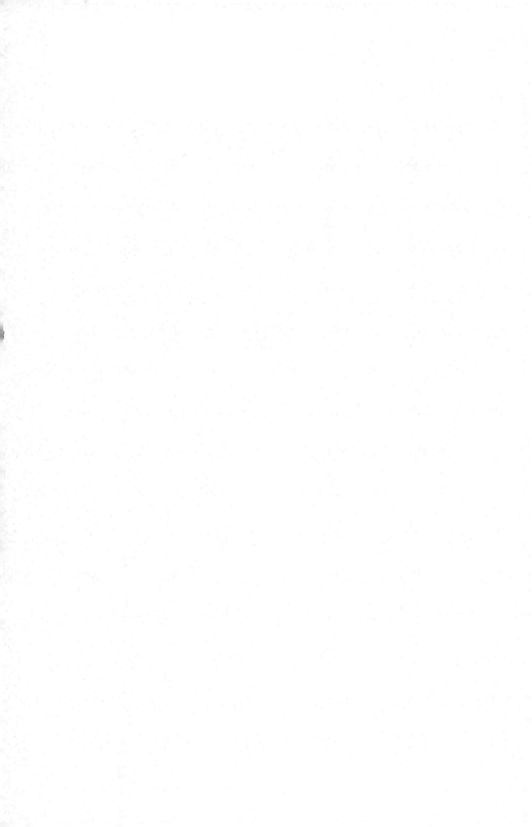

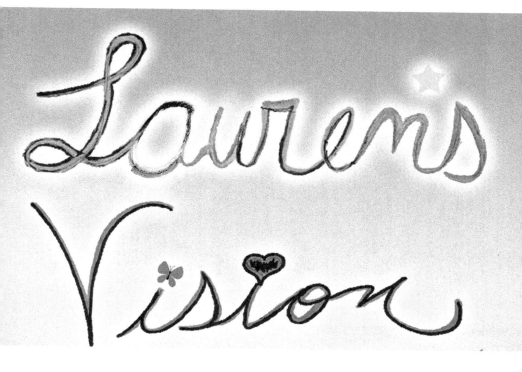

A Mother and Daughter's Journey of
Love, Loss and Learning to Live Again

E. LISA CUMMINS

Lauren's Vision

Library of Congress Cataloguing-in-Publication Data

E. Lisa Cummins, author

9798768114114 (paperback)

9798768104122 (hardcover)

9798784729606 (paperback large print)

9798784282095 (hardcover large print)

First Edition

Printed in the United States of America

The stories in this book reflect the author's recollection of events. Some names and organizations have been changed or initials used to protect the privacy of those depicted. Dialogue has been re-created from the author's journals and memories.

DEDICATION

For my daughter, Lauren, who is and will always be a symbol of light, beauty and love in this world.

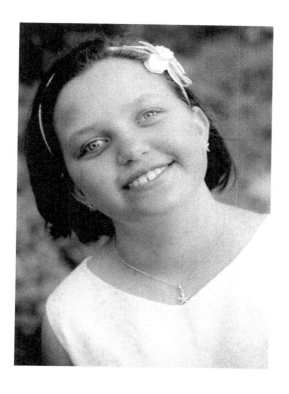

CONTENTS

FOREWORD

Writing a personal encounter about loss of a loved one is a monumental challenge. When combined with other significant losses, it becomes even more difficult. That's not to say this is a book solely about loss. It is so much more than that. The real focus is on love and living your best life despite trials and tribulations faced. I have had many of the same experiences as the author, and was so impressed by her tenacity, vulnerability, honesty and the way she always showed up for Lauren, and later for herself. I am honored to write the foreword for my friend and kindred spirit.

I first met Lisa in Miami at a Neuro-Linguistics Programming (NLP) practitioner certification training event in the spring of 2016. I was instantly drawn to her and when it was time to partner up for exercises, we found one another. We connected with a couple of other women who became our social and mastermind support during this intensive weekend and throughout the months of study ahead. Lisa and I quickly discovered it was no coincidence we were brought together. Our after class happy hours and dinner conversations became increasingly personal revealing we each had lost a child – a shared, unfathomable pain that knowing looks and holding hands across the table confirmed. When she mentioned she was working on writing Lauren's story, I shared the planning of my self-help book. We both felt that sharing our stories could help others. Another connection made. Before the weekend was over, Lisa confided concerns about her marriage, adding another layer to our talks. I had been through a difficult marriage and ultimately a

1

divorce, many years prior, which led me to becoming a professional life coach specializing in relationships.

In our time together, we recognized that we shared a love for learning and personal development. Part of my practice is facilitating workshops, seminars and support groups, and Lisa was being drawn to do the same. We both knew we were destined to work together as we grew our relationship both personally and professionally. It was not a matter of "if" but "when" and "what." I have no doubt that there will be other ventures one day, but for now, it is this very important work – Lauren's story, the one waiting to be told through Lisa's eyes.

For some, writing requires a creative process. But for Lisa, it was a combination of utilizing her project management expertise and book "coaching." As she recounted stories from her journals that helped her heal for years, she transferred them onto pages while structuring a timeline of Lauren's life like a manager. She referenced her organized spreadsheets and calendars from having managed Lauren's medical procedures to spark her memories and ensure she was authentic in the process. It was cathartic for her. No matter how many times you tell your own story, there is something very taxing and different about putting your story in writing. Revisiting all the experiences, both positive and negative, triggered emotional responses that Lisa had to sort. She had to bravely share some deep, inner truths and reflections that made her feel vulnerable from reopening wounds. She had to back away for a while. She visited friends and family. She rejuvenated. Many times she would have to restore her own soul, and then return to the book. She worried over small things, fretted over big things. In the fall of 2021, she came to visit me for a final read together. The manuscript was complete! We raised a glass to toast the completion of yet another milestone in her journey. She truly inspires admiration and wonder with all she has accomplished.

Lauren had a vision, and Lisa has graced us by sharing it. It's that simple and that complex. In doing so, Lisa speaks to us through her writing as if we are a friend by her side throughout. We connect to her, Lauren, Chris and others in the family, feeling the joy in their laughter and the pain in their sorrow. Lisa lets us into her intimate, personal space, opening herself to grow while using her truths to assist others. She shows us when we go through something so profound and arrive at the other side, we have a choice. We can focus on the pain and the wounds from the experience and live the rest of our life in that darkness, or we can acknowledge that it hurt like hell and that there were some amazingly feel good times, too. By focusing on the latter, she was able to keep her heart filled with love and allow the light to shine brightly for both herself and her beautiful daughter, Lauren.

The question to each of us becomes, *"Will you focus on the thorny stem or the rose?"* Lisa's journey during and beyond Lauren's earthly life takes her through a lot of thick, sharp, and pointed thorns, but she always manages to find the bloom among them. And by doing so, she inspires all of us to be able to do the same.

We will all see ourselves somewhere in this book.

— **Ann Papayoti**, CPC, Amazon bestselling author of two books, *Engaging Speakers Voices of Truth* and *The Gift of Shift*

INTRODUCTION

There are stories we tell ourselves about our life, how it is and what we expect it to be. We spend time worrying about things that never happen and get blown away by things that do. We are never ready for those life-altering moments that rock our world, leaving us to figure out how to pick up the pieces. We can find strength during these times, or we can fall apart. Sometimes we do both, which is only natural.

My tendency, which has also been one of my biggest challenges, is to be a "fixer". I analyze and overthink the situation, do what needs to be done to get back on track and collapse after. Somehow, I've always found the strength to pick myself up no matter how harrowing the situation. The problem is, there are things in life that cannot be fixed or even understood. What happened in my family would provide lesson after lesson that some things can't be controlled.

I was living the American dream. I had put myself through college, had professional success, bought a nice car and condo on the water, met a wonderful man and got married. We went on to have a family, move into our dream home and were getting all the things I thought we "deserved" and "should" do, be, and have. For a time, I got caught up in these superficial things. As curveballs and setbacks came my way, I learned to see past them. I realized life is about love, which transcends everything, including unimaginable loss and even the things we think of as boundaries, like time and distance.

I have come to understand that no matter when life comes to an end, love does not. My biggest lesson was realizing that love is not something to control or fear losing but rather something you give freely and carry with you always. It goes beyond the hurt of loss and our expectation of what is "supposed" to happen.

At its heart, this is a story about the depth and breadth of my immeasurable love for my child, the struggles we endured and the lessons we taught each other along the way. I had picked up the pen to write about my journey with Lauren many times, but life's trials and tribulations kept adding new pages and allowed me to see the old ones through a different lens. Maybe it took so long to finish this book because of the additional lessons I had to learn and process before I could write it in a way that would help others. Maybe I should have learned them sooner because my greatest teacher, my daughter Lauren, was all about love which is the core message that needs to be shared.

Even in her most challenging moments Lauren was concerned about others, always wanting to share her love and laughter. She took chances when I certainly wouldn't. She approached complete strangers when she felt like they needed support. She would give them one of her bracelets made out of pretty pastel-colored beads in the shape of stars, butterflies and hearts. To me, these shapes symbolized Lauren's light, beauty and love and personified who she was. To Lauren they represented something else. She'd say, "This bracelet has love, energy and power in every bead." They also served as a great conversation starter and a sure-fire way for her to engage with others.

There were times I wanted her not to "bother" anyone. But I watched and realized how wrong I was. Most people were lit up by my daughter's open, loving nature and to this day I meet people wearing those bracelets in stores, airports, beaches, all over the place – some can't put into words why they love their bracelet so much. Yet they all remember the little girl who gave it to them and the magic that comes from their bracelet.

It was easy to love Lauren, but by no means was it an easy life. It was filled with so many challenges and adversities, heartache, joy, loss, sadness and much more, but at its core, it was pure unconditional love. I wanted Lauren to know that no matter what she was loved, and that together we could get through anything. I was focused on loving Lauren unconditionally, but somewhere along the way I learned I was worthy and deserving of that, too. We all are. We just have to give our love away freely and expect nothing in return.

I admit, there were times when giving all I had to Lauren and my family, I lost touch with myself. That happens to so many mothers and caregivers. This journey has not only been about Lauren's challenges or the shocks that followed but also about loving myself, rediscovering who I am and reclaiming my own hopes and dreams. I'm living proof others can do the same.

I struggled with how much spiritual material I wanted to include in this book for fear of putting people off. But in my quest to help Lauren live her best life, I traveled down many unfamiliar paths because I did not want to leave any stone unturned. I was also willing to travel to the ends of the earth to try almost anything as long as it didn't hurt her and might help. We used Western and

Eastern medicine, meditation, alternative therapies and treatments, supplements and diets. I brought in spiritual healers, readers and teachers – some modalities people might consider pretty "out there." When I dive into those parts, take what you like and leave the rest. What I know for sure is all of this led me on a spiritual journey I never would have taken otherwise.

It's the spiritual part of my journey that taught me love stays with you always. I know this too, because I feel Lauren's love around me each and every day. She seems to have transcended death with her loving, positive ways and somehow encapsulated that in a bracelet. It has become a symbol of her love, energy and power that she embodied and goes on to lift others up and remind them that whatever life challenges they face, they got this. They realize, if Lauren can go through all she went through and live HPH (happy, positive and healthy), they can too. For me, Lauren taught me how precious life is and to live our best life every moment of every day. I could have never known at the time that all the love and strength I poured into her would come back to serve me in dealing with her loss and the aftershocks to come.

This is my tribute to my beautiful, sweet, kind, compassionate and amazing daughter – for the incredible life she lived and all those she touched – but most of all for her love.

Section One

LOVE

CHAPTER

One

Healthy Baby Girl

I'd been sitting in the hot waiting room for at least an hour with a squirming toddler in my lap and an infant in my arms. Needless to say, I was frustrated. Our doctor's office was spilling over with all kinds of people – young and old, poor and well-off. People came from all over to see Dr. L. He was holistic, adept in Western as well as Eastern medicine. He supported our choice not to vaccinate our children, and he had a great bedside manner: calm, gentle and soft-spoken. When the nurse finally called us in to see him, he was so pleasant I instantly forgot the annoying wait. "So sorry, Mrs. Cummins, next time we will get you in sooner."

My husband did most of the research to find Dr. L, whose office was not too far from where I worked and where our children attended a Montessori daycare program. We were impressed Dr. L traveled to China every year to study and stay up to date on the latest Eastern medicine practices, including acupuncture. I felt confident in him and proud to be on the cutting edge, having our babies cared for by a holistic practitioner.

My daughter Lauren, like her big brother Christopher, did fine at all her regular check-ups and hit all the milestones babies do. There was only one thing that worried me – from birth Lauren had spots all over her body – some big, some small. I asked Dr. L about them at almost every visit.

"You can tell just by looking at her that she is a healthy baby," he said each and every time.

She did look like a typical happy, healthy baby in spite of occasional fevers that were very high – around 104 – which was scary. I loved and watched my daughter grow and noted in her baby book what an independent little girl she was. At one year old she insisted on feeding herself and if her daycare teachers put her on her mat for a nap, she'd crawl away until she was ready. People who knew me joked, "I know where she gets it from."

Café-au-Lait

When Lauren was about two, something guided me to switch to a local pediatrician. I wanted someone closer to our house and an office where I wouldn't have to wait so long with two toddlers. Dr. L sometimes took us right away as a professional courtesy to my husband, who was a chiropractor at the time, but even so, it was becoming unmanageable.

I asked around at daycare for a pediatrician. There was a great network of moms and dads who used our company's onsite Montessori program. We would chat together, sharing information and advice as we dropped our kids off and walked to our offices in the main building. I found out about a pediatrician close to my home and when Lauren got a cold, that's when I decided to take her to this new doctor.

"Have you noticed these marks all over her body?" It was virtually the first thing the doctor said to me.

"Yes, I asked our doctor about them many times," I said.

"Has she been checked by a neurologist? Markings like these may be related to something, and it's best to have them checked," he said.

"A neurologist? Why? We noticed those birthmarks when she was born but she's always had a clean bill of health!" I told him. "No one ever recommended any type of follow-up – not at the hospital and not our doctor." I repeated what our doctor used to always say, "You can tell just by looking at her she is a healthy baby."

Those words echo in my mind to this day. I can't believe how Dr. L dismissed the markings over and over again. I trusted him, and of course, I wanted to believe there was nothing wrong with my baby girl. But I knew it – there were too many of these marks to be nothing.

"It's not urgent, but you should have her checked out to be on the safe side," the pediatrician told us. He gave me the name of a pediatric neurologist at Stony Brook University Hospital (SBUH). I made the appointment immediately, but it was an anxious month before they could see her.

The Diagnosis

The appointment with the pediatric neurologist was on a very cold day in February. After the exam, the doctor told us Lauren exhibited two out of seven symptoms of something called Neurofibromatosis Type 1, or NF1.

"Neuro-what?" I asked, stunned.

"NF1 is usually a genetic disorder. It can range from very mild to very severe. Lauren is only displaying two of the mildest symptoms, so I would say she has a mild case."

"So these markings on her body, they are one of the symptoms?" I asked.

"Yes, five or more light brown skin spots, 5 millimeters or bigger. They're called café au lait spots. French for coffee with milk."

"So, they aren't just beauty marks," I said. Lots of feelings were beginning to bubble up inside me. I could feel myself getting angry, but also felt a sense of guilt for not following my instincts. "What's the other symptom?"

"Lauren also has freckling under her arms and in her groin area," the doctor said.

"So these two symptoms mean she has NF1?"

"Yes, two or more of the seven possible symptoms confirms the diagnosis," he said.

He explained that NF1 is a chromosomal disorder, and if there is no family history, it is considered a genetic mutation. The other symptoms are far more severe, including tumors that can form anywhere in the nervous system, including the brain and spinal cord, scoliosis (curvature of the spine) and enlargement or deformation of the bones, such as bowing of the legs. Thankfully she didn't have any of these other symptoms, I thought to myself. But I was scared.

"Is there any family history of Neurofibromatosis?" the neurologist asked.

"No, not that we know of," I said, looking at my husband for confirmation. He looked as confused as I felt, then looked away.

After a moment, he confessed he'd suspected Neurofibromatosis when Lauren was a baby. "The data said it was genetic, so I dismissed it," he said.

"But you didn't say anything? You knew I wondered about all those marks! There were too many of them for it to be nothing!" I frantically said as I looked at him with bewildered eyes.

How could he *not* share that kind of information with me?

Letter Unsent

Now I was angry at my husband for not sharing his suspicions, at Dr. L for missing this diagnosis but also at myself for not taking Lauren for a second opinion when I questioned those markings to begin with. What had I done? Why didn't my husband share his concerns about something that serious so we could discuss it? I wondered what opportunities for early treatment or other information we might have missed. I resolved from that day forward I would always trust my mother's intuition.

I was very upset that our initial doctor missed such a serious diagnosis and clear symptoms and felt I had to do something. I decided to draft a letter and send it to Dr. L,

"....I have gone from disbelief to hysterics, from sad, to counting our blessings ....I can't help but wonder if this diagnosis was made earlier, we would have had the opportunity to do more research and monitor her more closely....I hope you realize the impact you have on children's lives and in the future you listen to a mother's concern and do not dismiss markings of this type."

"I don't think you should send that letter," my husband said.

"Why not? How could he not know about this?" I asked. "He was a doctor and he was supposed to know these things!"

"Doctors are human," he said.

I went back to this question over and over – for years. Every time Lauren's health would change and some other doctor didn't know what was going on, I would question how they could NOT know the answers.

I never did send that letter and was haunted by the thought that maybe if I had known sooner, I could have done something differently. The thought also occurred to me that maybe it was a blessing to have more time of pure joy and bliss, of just watching my daughter grow without concern that something was terribly wrong.

After Lauren's diagnosis, I alternated between relief and panic. Yes, Lauren's case of NF1 was mild now, but would it become debilitating later on? I would tell myself, "Lauren will grow up to have a happy, normal life!" But there was no way to know that for sure.

The neurologist told us we had to do two things right away: see an eye specialist and have Lauren assessed for scoliosis. The eye doctor would watch for optic-gliomas, which are growths on the optic nerve that could affect her vision. I didn't understand back then that this could possibly cause blindness, but I knew it was urgent to find a pediatric ophthalmologist, which I did right away. We had to wait another excruciating month for an appointment. As for the scoliosis, my husband was a chiropractor and had been giving adjustments to both Chris and Lauren since birth, so we knew there were no signs of that so far.

The neurologist also suggested we get genetic testing. A part of me wondered if one of us tested positive, would we feel blame or guilt? I know inheriting a disorder is nobody's fault, but when you're anxious and looking for answers, it's easy to forget what is rational and reasonable. We scheduled the test and waited.

CHAPTER

Two

Staying Normal

"Lauren has an astigmatism that we're going to correct with glasses," the eye specialist told us. It was just two days before Lauren's second birthday and this news was a relief. We took Lauren to get her very first pair of pink "Mickey" eyeglasses. I wished she could have perfect vision, but lots of little kids wore glasses, and to my surprise Lauren never gave us any trouble about wearing them. Watching Lauren make a beeline to her favorite yellow swing in our yard, she was the picture of a perfectly happy and healthy little girl who just happened to need pink Mickey Mouse glasses. She seemed to be taking them in stride. I was going to try to do the same.

I tend to always jump to worst-case scenarios and had to remind myself to breathe. When I got stressed about "what if?" scenarios, I also reminded myself Lauren didn't have serious symptoms – and the doctor said nothing else might ever develop. But I kept researching NF1 because I thought if I could understand it, maybe I could do something about it. The problem was this also fed my anxiety. When I am fearful and anxious, I can feel my body gearing up as if it is preparing for battle, latching up with a heavy coat of armor. My neck, shoulders and lower back all tight with tension. I was ready to fight for my baby girl and go into combat with NF1 and nothing would get in the way of that.

Knowledge is Power

There are two different types of Neurofibromatosis. NF1 is more common. Back in 1999 when Lauren was diagnosed, about one out of four thousand people in the United States had it. Since then, the statistics have changed to one in three thousand. So, either cases are on the rise, or more people are being diagnosed.

Symptoms of NF1, particularly café-au-lait spots or freckles on the skin, are often evident at birth or during infancy, and almost always appear by the time a child is about ten years old. Neuro-fibromas (tumors) become evident at around ten to fifteen years old. But that was a long time away and science could come up with a treatment by then. In most cases, symptoms are mild and patients live normal and productive lives. In some cases, however, NF1 can be severely debilitating. I wanted to think positive – Lauren would be one of the lucky ones and never develop any more symptoms, and if not, by that time there'd be a cure.

Although many people inherit NF1, between thirty and fifty percent of new cases are caused by spontaneous mutation in utero. Once this happens, there is a fifty percent chance of passing the condition on. I thought about Lauren eventually passing NF1 to her children. Maybe she would choose not to have a baby. Would my little girl get to have that amazing experience when she grew up?

When we finally got the genetic test results back, we found neither one of us carried the gene, so Lauren's case was considered a genetic mutation. While these results didn't change the fact that Lauren had NF1, it did stop my ruminating thoughts about the possibility that one of us may have passed it on to her and how it might have ultimately affected our relationship.

It was very strange to feel both relieved and frightened at the same time. Regardless, managing and coping with my daughter's health issues became my new normal. I just wanted us to be a regular family, but I would stay on alert for anything that might be off with Lauren.

Slightly Behind

When I found out that fifty percent of children with NF1 are susceptible to developmental and learning delays, I remembered that Lauren's lead teacher at daycare felt Lauren was slightly behind the other children in her class. There was no real reason for concern up until the diagnosis, but now I had to see if she was delayed. And if so, was it was related to NF?

"Why are you looking for things to be wrong with her?" my husband asked me. "She doesn't have learning disabilities!"

It felt like he was accusing me of something, and it raised some tension between us. I could not make him understand why I was being so cautious. I was just not willing to let any other symptom go unchecked, especially after not following up on my suspicions of the café-au-lait marks. I scheduled an evaluation in spite of his protests.

It took two months to finish all the testing. When we finally got the results, we found out that Lauren's hearing was fine, but she had delays in speech as well as in her fine and gross motor skills. She would require occupational, speech and physical therapy.

We both now realized how important it was not to let anything else slip by us. I get that it's hard for a parent to think there is something wrong with their child. It's easy to slip into denial. But I had a "not on my watch," policy. Nothing else was going to go unchecked. If there was anything I could control about my child's future health, I was determined to do it.

Two Wolves

After a few physical therapy sessions, the therapist pointed out that Lauren seemed to be slightly bow-legged and that she locked her knees.

"It could be developmental, something she'll just outgrow," he said.

"Well, I'm not willing to take any chances," I said. It was another symptom of NF1 and now with my husband on board, it was easier to make sure Lauren got whatever she needed as early as possible.

We were fortunate that I had great medical benefits through my company and could get Lauren the best doctors. Unfortunately, the most highly recommended pediatric orthopedist didn't take any insurance. But if he was the best, we didn't care how much it cost. I was surprised when we arrived at his small, outdated office.

"This is the office of a top doctor?" I thought to myself.

Dr. P came in wearing black leather pants and a casual T-shirt. He had funky curly black hair and a kid-friendly approach. After examining Lauren, he told us that her legs would more than likely self-correct.

"She's two, and children at her age tend to overcorrect and then straighten out," he said. He saw how concerned we were about her NF1 diagnosis. While we let Lauren play in the waiting room, he told us a story that has always stayed with me.

"In all my years, I've only treated two other children with the same diagnosis as Lauren. Both their families wanted to make the best possible choices for them. One family decided to keep on living their life as normally as they could. They worked and stayed together. The other parents, both lawyers, quit their jobs and relocated to be near the best hospital they could find."

Now, I thought this was the family he would say did the right thing. I was all on board with that, ready to agree with him. We would do the same thing, I thought. I'd move heaven and earth for my child, pay any price and go to extreme lengths to get Lauren what she needed.

But the doctor continued, "They spent their life savings, turned their lives upside-down and ended up getting divorced. The children both had the same outcome, but one family was together and the other wasn't. One was much happier and more stable than the other. Keep your routine as much as possible for the sake of everyone."

Now I understood what he was trying to tell us. Keep life normal. Don't focus on the illness and make yourselves crazy because it can tear you apart. Get your child the care they need, but consider the impact your decisions will have on the family.

"I get it," I said, but it was hard.

His philosophy reminded me of a Cherokee Indian story that goes: An old Cherokee was teaching his grandson about life. "A fight is going on inside me," he said to the boy. "It is a terrible fight, and it is between two wolves. One is evil. He is filled with anger, envy, sorrow, regret, greed, arrogance, self-pity, guilt, resentment, inferiority, lies, false pride, superiority and ego."

"The other is good. He is filled with joy, peace, love, hope, serenity, humility, kindness, benevolence, empathy, generosity, truth, compassion and faith. The same fight is going on inside you – and inside every other person, too."

The grandson thought about it for a minute and then looked at his grandfather and asked, "Which wolf will win?"

The old Cherokee replied, "The one you feed."

I had to decide which wolf I was going to feed and which family we were going to be.

Family Fun and Traditions

Sometimes on the way home, I'd be tired, burnt out from a long day at work, and just wanting to kick off my shoes and relax, but we'd pass the park on Pond Path and the kids would beg me to stop. They called it the Choo-Choo Train Park because of the jungle gym shaped like a train engine. I'd cringe at the thought of another half hour before I could get out of my office attire, but then Lauren would spot the swings, and sometimes the Mr. Softee truck was there as an added enticement. There were times I said no, but I am glad for every time I said, "Ok, but just for a little while," because today, I get to remember how they both loved it there.

Another way we kept things "normal" was to stay close to our families. Since I lived so close to my sister, Marion, we would hang out a lot on weekends and do fun things and have many family dinners together. Marion has four children and her two youngest, Julianne and Kelcie, were close in age to Chris and Lauren. We both enrolled our girls in dance classes and Lauren loved everything about it. She loved the music and socializing with other girls her age. She especially loved the recitals at the end of each year and dressing up in beautiful dance costumes.

My family also had an all-day family reunion every summer at Lido Beach. It was a place where all my aunts, uncles and cousins would meet up. There was a park with swings, a kiddie pool and splash area that Lauren loved. We also had the beach and ocean. My dad loved to play horseshoes with his brothers, sons and sons-in-law, and the whole family would participate in beach volleyball. It was always a great day of family fun!

On my husband's side, we attended a massive annual family reunion in quaint Williamstown, NY. Every February, we'd pile in the car and drive to the Carmelite Retreat Center. The rooms were small and simple with brick walls, tile floors, a bed and an end table. The only decoration was a cross hanging over the door. One room at the end of the hall unfortunately backed onto an indoor basketball court.

25

We all prayed not to get that room because balls thudded against those walls night and day. We'd ski and go snow-tubing and shop in the nearby town. Best of all was gathering at the end of the day in the common room where a big fire would be roaring and drinks would be flowing. Then this very Irish family would get up and show off their talents, which included step dancing, singing and dancing. And cousin Steven would perform his version of "bacon" – where he would get down on the floor and move his body starting out slow, then move faster and faster, like a piece of bacon cooking on the stove. Chris showed off his breakdancing and the little cousins, including Lauren, would run around in circles. The rest of us just laughing and taking it all in.

On the last morning, we would attend mass in the small on-site chapel. Uncle John would always pray for Lauren.

Dear Father in Heaven,
We thank you for this beautiful weekend and gathering of our family. We thank you for the food, laughter and fun we experienced together. We thank you for all your love and goodness and ask that you send your healing light to our Lauren and keep her well. Amen.

It was traditions like these that allowed us to stay close to both our families. Though we got to see my family more often because of how close we lived and because we had kids the same age, we made sure we alternated holidays that allowed us to have family bonds.

The love, strength and support of our families was essential for allowing us to keep things normal. This was something I never thought I would ever have to doubt.

CHAPTER

Three

Pitiful Or Powerful

That fall, Lauren developed bronchitis that wouldn't go away. We thought it might be pertussis and were very worried. We were faced with confronting the fact we hadn't vaccinated the kids, which was a little controversial, and wondered if we had we done the right thing? While I agreed to take the more holistic route regarding our children's health, now given Lauren's condition I was reconsidering that decision. When we went to the doctor, Lauren got an antibiotic and we talked to him about vaccinating her when her cough cleared up. I felt we had to protect her every way we could.

I had to keep reminding myself the reasons why we did this. Since Chris and Lauren weren't vaccinated as infants, they'd had a chance to build up their immune systems. Plus, I breastfed them until they were well over a year old. Surely, they had a big advantage from all that.

High Alert

I want to say I didn't hyper-focus on Lauren's condition and our lives didn't revolve around it, but looking back it's clear how much time and energy the situation demanded. We were alternating visits between Lauren's ophthalmologist and neurologist every six months, so she was always seeing a specialist. Lauren was also getting OT, PT and speech at daycare. And I was the one coordinating all of those appointments and therapy sessions while managing my demanding job with its hectic meetings and deadlines.

I was worried and stressed over all that was going on and felt like I was always on alert. I would go over to daycare often to check on Lauren and to meet with her therapists. Lauren seemed to take all of this in stride. To her and her brother, nothing was wrong or unusual. Lauren just had some additional teachers (therapists) to play with her one-on-one and went to the doctor when she needed to and that was that. There was still lunch with mom in the cafeteria, which they both loved, and visits to my desk to say hi to my co-workers.

Now What?

The time for Lauren's six-month appointment with the eye doctor rolled around and we expected a routine follow up. The worst we imagined was that she might need new glasses. I was at my desk when the phone rang that Thursday afternoon.

"The doctor is going to dilate her eyes. I think you should come over here right away," my husband said.

I flew out of the office and made it there in record time. I found Lauren and her daddy sitting in the waiting room.

"We're waiting for her pupils to dilate," he said.

Before he could say anything else, the nurse called us in. Now the doctor could see Lauren's optic nerves.

"I don't like the way her left optic nerve looks," he said. "It should be bright pink but it's pale. We need to run some more tests."

The nurse in the room stuck out her hand to Lauren. "Let's go play in the waiting room!" she said.

"Now what?" my husband asked the doctor.

"I want to schedule an MRI to have a brain scan," the doctor said. "It looks like she's lost vision in her left eye." He didn't sugarcoat anything.

"She lost her vision? How is that possible?" I asked. "It's only six months since she was here!" I felt myself floating away. I couldn't even listen anymore. My husband grabbed my hand and squeezed. How could I have missed something like my child completely losing vision in one eye? But Lauren was only two and half years old. She couldn't tell me if her vision had changed. We were dependent on the doctor's instruments.

The eye doctor called the neurologist for us, and Lauren was scheduled for an MRI in a month. It turns out we didn't have to wait for that appointment. Over the weekend Lauren complained that her head hurt. When I called the doctor, he said she needed an emergency MRI. It was the first of many times I would hear that phrase. I sat with Lauren in the back seat stroking her hair as we raced to the hospital.

As soon as we arrived, three interns surrounded her. They gave her a sedative and I held her in my arms until she fell asleep. Over and over I whispered, "Everything is going to be okay." It was more for my benefit than hers.

"Can you put a blanket on her to keep her warm?" I asked when it came time for the scan.

I watched from a tiny square window as my little girl was swallowed up in the MRI tube. I was both frustrated and terrified because she was only two and half years old and I couldn't be in the room with my baby. What if she woke up and needed me? When a technician finally appeared in the waiting area, I raced over to him.

"We need to take another scan, this time with contrast," he said.

Lauren would need two more injections. The nurse pulled her out of the machine to inject more sedative and contrast. The shots immediately woke her up and she started screaming. We could not settle Lauren down, much less get her back to sleep. Fortunately, the radiologist called, saying he had good images after all. I was relieved and furious that my baby was so traumatized. I calmed her down just as the neurologist walked in, bringing three other doctors with him. He didn't pull any punches.

"The diagnosis is bi-lateral optic gliomas. The left optic nerve is infiltrated by the glioma. It reaches all the way back to the chiasm, where the optic nerves cross. A small portion of the right optic nerve is also affected."

For me, these words were essentially a blur.

"What does that mean?" we asked.

"She has growths – possibly tumors - on both of her optic nerves."

"Oh my God." I felt like a fog was rolling in. Though his lips were moving, the doctor's voice got fainter and farther away.

"I'll be fading out at this point and turning Lauren's case over to the head of pediatric oncology," he said.

"What? Why?" I asked, my eyes stinging with tears.

"I don't understand!" I said to him. "One minute you are Lauren's main doctor and now we are being passed to someone we don't even know! What is happening?"

He didn't answer.

"Why oncology, does she have cancer?" I looked back and forth from my husband to the neurologist.

"The oncologist will give you more information. He'll have a protocol for treatment," the neurologist said. Then he walked away. We just stood there for a little while in complete silence.

I was numb. I don't remember the drive home, whether we talked or I cried, whether Lauren slept or fussed. I shut down and this was unlike me. I obsessed over what all this meant for Lauren. It made me sick to my stomach and emotionally paralyzed to the point I could not move. I was unable to do any normal tasks or household items. I was lost in the worst-case scenarios and frozen by the thought this thing could take Lauren from me. While she and Christopher spent the weekend playing, I curled up into a ball on the couch and didn't move unless I had to throw up.

It must have been Wednesday morning. Three days since the MRI. I woke up feeling someone's eyes on me. Christopher was standing over me. "Mommy? Are you OK?" he asked with my husband watching.

"Lisa, you can't stay on the couch forever," my husband said softly to me.

In that moment I realized that both my babies needed me. It was time to get up. One of my favorite quotes from author and bible teacher Joyce Meyer is, "You can be pitiful or powerful, pick one." I decided in that moment to be powerful and to pick myself up and get going.

There was work to be done and things to organize, which is one of my strengths. As a program manager for a large IT company, that skill set would serve me well. Lists, charts and excel spreadsheets were my friends. They gave me a sense of order and accomplishment. So, I created Lauren's notebook to keep a record of everything I found out about her condition. I created spreadsheets for doctors and therapists, to show our research and observations about how Lauren was doing each day. Without those notes, I wouldn't be able to tell you what the doctor said back then. I also starting journaling more to help me cope and write about my feelings.

There was still plenty I didn't understand, so I trusted that since my husband was a chiropractor and had taken biology and anatomy, he would explain what I didn't understand. What he didn't know, he would ask or look up later.

Chemo

When we met with the oncologist, he recommended Lauren start chemotherapy right away. That's a word you never want to hear, especially when it relates to your child.

"We want a second opinion," I said. There was no way we were making this kind of decision here and now.

The top specialist for NF1 tumors in Washington, D.C. was the doctor who'd founded the protocol the oncologist had recommended. We immediately flew out to meet him and he agreed that chemotherapy would be Lauren's best option.

"Lauren has a 'low-grade' malignancy," he told us. "We've had good results with two drugs in combination, vencristine and carboplatin."

Only God's grace allowed me to be calm and curious instead of panicked and terrified. No one had used the term "malignancy" up until now. The other doctor called the tumor "benign."

Here we were, two parents who didn't even believe in vaccinations and now we had to put toxic chemicals into our daughter's little body?

"How long is the treatment?" I asked.

"The typical length for this chemo is 18 months," the doctor said.

"Eighteen *months*?" I said. "What about her beautiful blonde hair?"

It might seem like a trivial thing, but I had to ask. Was I shallow to think about how people can stare? Was it silly to worry that other kids would be mean to Lauren if her hair fell out? Wasn't getting better the only important thing? Maybe, but with the world swirling, it seemed to me like that little thing mattered too.

The following week we saw the oncologist back on Long Island. He said there were three options. The first was to watch and hope the tumor didn't grow. But there was evidence it already was growing. Plus, her ophthalmologist confirmed she had no light perception in her left eye and the vision in the right eye could also decline. Doing nothing was out.

The second option was to perform surgery and remove the tumor. "The operation would completely blind her," the oncologist said.

"Most of the time with an NF1 tumor on the optic nerve, it will impair vision but stop growing by age six," he said. If there was hope that could happen, we weren't in favor of removing the tumor and risk her losing her vision entirely.

The third option was chemo. Lauren had already lost vision in her left eye and chemotherapy would help preserve the vision in her right.

"It's the best option considering the alternatives," he said. After hearing all three options, chemo seemed to be the one that made the most sense and we agreed to move forward.

Lauren had her first surgery to have a mediport implanted in her chest to make IV treatments easier and began her chemo treatments a month later. It was the beginning of the Christmas season and instead of picking a tree, we were watching our child go through "induction" where she would get blasted with chemo before getting time off for her body to recover and start the standard frequency. Lauren's induction period would be chemo once a week for four weeks and then two weeks off. This would be our holiday season.

I did my best to continue to keep things normal, including our holiday traditions. Lauren liked to help me set up our Christmas village and nativity and, of course, making holiday cookies at Aunt Marion's with her cousins. I think she mostly loved eating the batter and the warm cookies and whatever other treats my sister would slip her. "Hey Aunt Marion, got anything else for me," she would say, thinking I couldn't hear or see her.

Divide and Conquer

After the New Year, Lauren started the standard protocol: chemo once a week for three weeks and then one week off so she could recover. Luckily, she didn't have many side effects. If she got nauseous, the anti-nausea medication usually did the trick. She didn't lose her hair, but it did thin out – a constant reminder to me of everything she was going through.

Hospital days were hard. Lauren went on Fridays because she would get tired from her treatments and needed the weekend to recover. I went for the first several treatments so I could have a good understanding of what was happening, and after that she went with her daddy. I would visit during my lunchtime and would have loved to stay with her the whole day, but we relied on my job for the income and medical benefits. It broke my heart not to be there, but we had to develop a "divide and conquer" approach to accomplish everything that had to get done.

"Mommy!" Lauren would shout when she saw me coming in with lunch. Her eyes would open bright, and I'd go over to kiss her hello.

"How's my baby girl?"

"Great!" Then I'd get to hear about all the silly things her daddy did to torment the nurses, including rolling his chair across the floor while yelling, "Watch out!" He loved being the center of attention and the infusion room gave him a captive audience. Lauren used to say that one of his jobs was to make her laugh. It made me happy to see her laugh, and it was hard not to laugh right along with her. Sometimes laughter is the best medicine!

I was the more serious one. My job was to not only be the doting mom but also be the squeaky wheel and make sure my little girl had everything she needed and I did just that. The mom in me put taking care of my girl first and foremost. I didn't care if I didn't seem like the fun one. Nothing was going to stop me from taking care of business for my girl. At times when opinions differed, we'd just agree to disagree. We both knew we had Lauren's best interest at heart and had different ways of showing it.

Nutrition is another area we focused on. We read books and met with nutritionists. From this, we learned to limit sugar and increase raw foods. We started incorporating things like wheatgrass into Lauren's diet which was high in nutrients and antioxidants. No matter what we did to make these green drinks delicious, Lauren would say, "This is not a yummy smoothie!" It wasn't easy to get a three year old to eat healthy all the time because not everything tasted good, but we did our best and so did Lauren.

The more we read and met with nutritionists, the more we were exposed to other holistic approaches to health. We met people who offered their knowledge and a variety of supplements, from powders to pills. They all claimed to cure diseases, including cancer. We wanted to be careful not to give Lauren anything that would conflict with the chemo and always spoke to her doctor before giving her anything. There was a fascinating world of holistic approaches to well-being out there and we were both open and ready to learn about and try whatever we could. I was especially willing to do whatever it took to keep my girl healthy and rid her of this tumor or at least keep it at bay.

Outta Here

After fifteen months of chemo, an MRI showed the tumor was no longer growing. The doctors said it was okay to stop treatment and just observe her. On her last day of chemo, we brought lunch for the doctors and nurses and had a big cake that said, "I'm Outta Here!" Everyone cheered for this little girl who had become a champion of being happy and positive despite all the poking and prodding of needles and IVs she had to endure.

Easter was early that year. The Cummins' annual family reunion was right before the holiday. Lauren's grandma, whom she called Mammie, brought up a beautiful pastel green Easter dress to give to Lauren for her fourth birthday. She immediately wanted to try it on, and I will never forget how beautiful Lauren looked, twirling like a princess. "Look at me, Mammie!" she said. It didn't matter that her

37

hair had completely thinned out from chemo. When she smiled, her big blue eyes lit up as she showed off her new dress.

We spent Easter with my family and thanked God Lauren had finished her treatment. The tumor hadn't grown – though it hadn't shrunk either – and the doctors felt the chemo had done its job. We were out of the woods and now our lives could go back to normal.

"Normal" had grown to include relying on family. Whenever I needed someone to watch Chris, I dropped him off at Marion's, who lived ten minutes from Stony Brook University Hospital. Marion and her husband Jeff became a second mom and dad to my guys – and our kids were more like siblings than cousins. Jeff would often tease Lauren and tell her to call him Oh Great One or OG1 for short.

"Ok OG1, but just so you know, that means Old Grey One!" Lauren would say with a twinkle in her eye and little giggle and grin she would always make.

Lauren always loved their house because they had two black labs, Barkley and Wisdom, that she played with. My sister also had plenty of delicious snacks and candy, which you could not find at our house. As usual, Marion would continue to slip Lauren treats when I wasn't looking.

"Hey Aunt Marion, what do you have for me?" Lauren whispered as Marion slipped her some Swedish Fish or potato chips. She also showed Lauren a drawer where she kept gum, breath mints and change and told Lauren she could help herself anytime...and she would!

It was a blessing to come from such big families and be able to count on their help whenever we needed them. Love surrounded my little girl. Each family member had a very special relationship or "thing" with Lauren.

My mom loved to garden and often came out with plants to do some gardening with me and Lauren. She got her green thumb from her mom (my Oma – German for Grandma) and so the love of gardening has been passed from mother to daughter, which I passed on to Lauren. My baby girl always loved to help however she could. There was something so peaceful to be out in nature listening to the birds and bringing beauty to our yard.

"Mommy, can we plant some pink flowers this year?"

Lauren had three favorite colors and would say why she loved them: yellow for "sunshine," red for "love" and pink for "pinky." I'm not sure what that last one meant but it was just one of the goofy little things she said. I think she loved pink because it was such a "girly girl" color. So, our garden always included those colors.

Lauren also loved to talk to the nurses at the hospital about their favorite colors and their families. She especially loved talking to the younger nurses and asking them questions about their boyfriends. She won the hearts of everyone with her positivity and charm. Even the nurses at pre-surgical that she only got to see once in a while remembered her. One nurse in particular adored Lauren and always called her "My Lau Lau."

One thing for sure is that Lauren always knew how to make people smile and left a powerful impression on others! No matter how many challenges this child endured, she carried an innate and uncanny ability to bring sunshine everywhere she went.

CHAPTER
Four

Making Wishes

Before we left the hospital, Lauren's oncologist told us he had a nice surprise for us.

"For once!" I joked. I couldn't imagine what he was talking about.

"Lauren has been granted a wish from the Make-A-Wish Foundation."

I was a little confused by this.

"I thought that was only for kids who were terminally ill," I said.

"No, it's for children who have life-threatening or critical illnesses and I referred her for a wish. Lauren has been through a lot; you all have. She should have a wish granted and it's time for all of you to have some fun!"

Part of my confusion was that I never really considered Lauren sick or as having a critical illness. Yes, she was having chemo, but I

41

looked at her needing these treatments as a precautionary measure to shrink down what was described as a "benign" tumor. After all, she had NF1 not *cancer*, and these types of tumors typically stop growing by age six. The worst we were told could happen was that it would impair her vision. This is what I remember being told to me over and over again, or at least what I thought I heard.

"I don't really feel comfortable accepting a trip from Make a Wish," I said. "There are so many deserving children out there, and we aren't struggling financially or anything, and Lauren is going to be fine."

The doctor repeated, "It's for children and their families to enjoy themselves after everything they have been through. You should at least consider it," he said.

I reluctantly agreed and soon after, two "Wish Granters" came to our house to talk to Lauren.

"If you could have any wish at all, what would it be? You can go anywhere or meet anyone you want." They said to her.

"I want to go to Disney so I can meet the princesses," she answered right away. She got her wish and the icing on the cake was that Mammie and Pop Pop would be coming along too.

Wish Trip

The first-class treatment started the minute we landed in Orlando and Make-a-Wish volunteers met us at the gate. They gave us a car and sent us off to Give Kids the World (GKTW), where we'd be staying. This is a non-profit resort primarily operated by volunteers who host Make-a-Wish families visiting Disney World.

I was surprised that it was an all-volunteer staff who made these memorable experiences possible for families. It touched my heart and also Christopher's. Many years later, we would go back as a family to volunteer, and Chris would continue to do so throughout college as well.

On our Disney Day, Lauren proudly wore her big pink "Wish" button, which signaled the Disney staff members and characters at the park to do whatever they could to make the visit magical. It also let us use the Fast Pass lanes! Lunch with the characters and all the princesses at Cinderella's Magical Castle was truly Lauren's dream come true. I was awed by the generosity of everyone at Give Kids the World and Disney. It dawned on me how much of an ordeal we'd all been through, just like the other families we met whose child got to Make-a-Wish. We all had something in common; and now we had a village designed to make them happy. Just kids and their families and everyone's wish was for them to be like any other child and have fun.

It truly took a "Village" to help me relax, get perspective on my child's journey and to rediscover my gratitude for generosity and kindness. My eyes were open to strangers who serve with no thought of return. I remembered how blessed I felt and how grateful I was for my family, especially my daughter, who was able to enjoy this amazing trip.

First Healing Touch

When we got home, a colleague at work told me about his relative, Bill, who was a scientist that developed a pill he believed cured his wife's breast cancer. He encouraged me to reach out to him and see if there was anything that could help Lauren.

We met with Bill, and he felt a supplement he developed could help Lauren. He went on to tell us something a little unorthodox. He said that in working with patients he began to feel vibration and heat in his hands, and he would place them on the person's back for a period of time. He felt this "placing of hands" seemed to assist in the healing process. I knew very little about energy healing at that time, but that is exactly what he was describing. The fact that he was a scientist and his own admission that this sounded a little crazy, gave us the confidence to be willing to try it. After a period of time, there were no significant results. As a man of science, Bill proposed that we stop. We were disappointed, but it would not be the last time we would try healing touch or other modalities that would be very new and different to us.

I needed stress relief and started going to meditation classes with an amazing teacher who offered guided meditation and workshops. When I was pregnant, I learned the Bradley Method, which taught me breathing techniques to help with labor and delivery. When I took meditation classes it reminded me of the same feeling of relaxation. Meditation resonates deeply and has always called to me. Even though Chris was six and Lauren was four, I started taking them to meditation classes too. My meditation teacher suggested that Lauren do affirmations. Lauren took to the practice quickly and enjoyed saying them out loud with conviction:

"I am healthy! I am strong! I am powerful!"

At the end of each meditation, we were given the opportunity to write about or share our experience with the group. During this time of reflection, I was able to re-center myself and feel a peace and calm I had not felt in a long time. I realized I had to take more time for myself and also needed to make time for my relationship with my husband.

Letters From the Heart

Romance had been missing from my relationship for a while now and I wished we had more time for it. There was a lot of focus over the last four years on Lauren with everything she was going through which was totally understandable, at least for me. On the occasions when I tried to make things special and nice for us, I was often disappointed by my husband's lack of emotion and affection. When he did show affection, it felt contrived. He portrayed being loving when others were around, but when we were alone, he pulled away. He seemed distant and emotionally unavailable, but it wasn't the first time.

As I thought about this, I flashed back to the time after we got engaged and discovered he secretly drank heavily. He had hidden this well and I was surprised to find out that his family already knew. I told him that I could not be with him if this is what life would be like. I had seen the toll my father's drinking took on my parent's marriage and did not want this to be a part of my life. He swore he would stop drinking and would get help. It wouldn't be until a few months after we were married, that I would find out even with all the support he was getting, he never stopped. It was at that point he decided to go

45

to a thirty-day rehab and I spent a month as a newlywed alone in bed wondering what things would be like when he returned. Would the drinking really stop this time? Or would there be more secrets?

During this period, he wrote me letters from the heart. We both went to counseling individually and as a couple and our relationship grew stronger. I was excited for our future and was looking forward to starting a family. We made lots of adjustments which included no alcohol in the house, at family gatherings or going to bars. While I was thrilled that the drinking seemed to finally stop, it came at a cost. He seemed to be less emotionally expressive and affectionate to me than he was before. We decided to travel and have some fun. From there, things seemed to get back on track. To my knowledge, he never drank again – I could not have imagined that one day he'd simply substitute one vice for another.

Getting back to where we are in this story, I attributed his emotionally pulling back now to the strain of everything we were going through. It was heartbreaking, to say the least, to watch Lauren endure vision loss, fifteen months of chemo and endless doctor visits and therapy treatments. A relationship can really suffer with so much stress and pressure from caring for a child with health issues. I assumed that once things were better with Lauren, we would get back on track as husband and wife again.

Time For Us

Our tenth wedding anniversary was coming up. With Lauren's chemo behind us, it seemed like a perfect time to get away and reconnect like I wished for. I started looking for something spectacular we could do together to mark this special milestone on so many counts. Lauren and Chris were both doing well, and the worst seemed to be behind us.

I found a river rafting trip down the Grand Canyon that looked incredible and normally had a year-long wait. I was thrilled when I found out that one of the tours had a cancellation the week of our anniversary. It felt as if it was meant to be. It would be the first time since both kids were born that we went away on vacation without them. Chris was now six and Lauren was four. I was nervous about leaving them, and even more so when I realized that we would have no cell service while at the base of the canyon. Mammie and Pop Pop offered to stay at our house for the week and take care of the kiddos, so we decided to go and just do it.

Shooting Star

Sleeping under the stars at the bottom of the Grand Canyon made me feel like a speck in a vast universe as I looked up at a black velvet sky filled with sparkling diamonds. On the evening of our anniversary, our new canyon friends decided they would help us renew our vows. They made me a bouquet of sticks and canyon flowers and one of the river rafters played his guitar while the lead guide officiated the ceremony to celebrate our ten years together.

We laughed and danced – and there was my husband, the center of attention again, but this time with me by his side. Afterward, as we walked back to our sleeping bags, he dropped my hand and walked ahead. I was used to it and chalked it up to his inability to fully express his feelings. Anyway, I was content with our rustic vow renewal. To cap the night, we saw a shooting star. Even though we weren't connecting one hundred percent, I believed it meant something: a blessing on our anniversary and our future.

After the trip, I have to admit, I was almost a little jealous of these river rafters who could detach from the real world and be transported to the beauty at the bottom of the canyon and just be one with nature for weeks at a time. It was so calming, relaxing, as well as exciting. I was grateful for my time in the canyon, walking her trails and riding her rapids while feeling so incredibly small yet part of something much larger. I didn't want to lose the awe I felt or the feeling of connection of my body to the earth. I felt my spirit was at ease for the first time in so long. I wanted to hold on to those feelings for as long as I could. I talked about all of this in my meditation classes when we were encouraged to use our imaginations to transport ourselves to a peaceful place. For a long time, mine was the majestic Grand Canyon.

Leaning Forward

Meditation was such a beautiful way to connect body, mind and spirit and a wonderful outlet for me. As I deepened my practice and studies, I continued to learn about many different holistic techniques and treatments to pursue my dream of finding something, anything, that would help my daughter. Once I opened my mind, I met person after person with information about some incredible method or approach. There were times I wondered whether to introduce some of the things I was learning about into Lauren's treatment. I talked

48

it over with my husband. We agreed if something didn't hurt Lauren and could possibly help her, we were willing to consider it.

I've heard it said many times that: "Life can only be understood looking backwards; but must be lived forwards." Looking back even at this point, I can see how this applied to much that was happening and how I was being prepared for what was yet to come. We have no way of knowing how things that happen to us will fit into the grand plan for our life. Simple things like a new breathing or healing technique can be a powerful soul-saving gift while other clear signposts get overlooked.

Life-Changing Speakers

I was happy my husband and I were both working and contributing toward creating our best life. I was the saver and planner; he was the spender and spontaneous. I'd been working full-time since I was seventeen and looked forward to the day when I wouldn't have to work anymore and could just spend time enjoying my family and all life had to offer.

My corporate job came with many demands, creating a lot of pressure. It also required me to travel periodically. The dream of someday leaving the corporate world to discover my own passion is what drew me to a book about creating multiple streams of income. When I read that the authors offered a weekend seminar, I decided to go. The event was held in November in Florida. I went with a co-worker. I was intrigued by three very different speakers who would change my life forever.

The first speaker was an ex-chiropractor who created a method of investing in the stock market. He developed a course on his proven

49

system. Since I loved numbers and managing money, I was all in on this one and signed up for his class. I never quite became an options trader, but it gave me a love of the stock market and taught me how to maximize my investments.

Next was a man who called himself a "Pranic Healer." He explained that Pranic Healing is an ancient energy healing technique that taps into *prana* or *ki* or vital energy to heal the whole person: physically, emotionally and mentally. He told us how he used this hands-on energy healing to help his wife, who'd been in a horrible accident, to expedite her healing. The results amazed the doctors. He had students all over the country. He did a live demonstration of this energy healing work on everyone in the room, and we all felt it. It was so impressive, that as soon as I got home, I found the closest Pranic Healer and took Lauren to see him. I also signed up for a workshop to learn how to use the technique myself.

The third speaker, and person that would have the biggest impact on our lives, was well known. He'd written a book about having a "wealth mindset" and created his own company to offer workshops. He offered a free three-day seminar that was about more than just money. It included proven ways to manage your money effectively and create financial opportunities for more income. It also taught you how to overcome any limiting thoughts, beliefs and feelings that keep you from the wealth, health, abundance and freedom you deserve and desire in this life – all while living a mindful life with integrity. This man had a boastful swagger that bordered on arrogant, but I found him likable. I was intrigued and took two free tickets to his event and planned on attending.

I was excited and hopeful that my wish for our family to have a future filled with health, happiness and prosperity would come true!

CHAPTER

Five

Broken Heart

My dad's heart broke for Lauren (and for me) when she had to go through chemo. He told me many times that he would have given his life for her. Though he never stopped drinking altogether, my dad mellowed so much and opened up more and more as he got older. I know he loved his family, but as kids we never knew what we were going to get when he walked through the door. When he drank, he was either really happy and the life of the party or super nasty, like Dr. Jekyll and Mr. Hyde. When he wasn't drinking, he was quiet and emotionally withdrawn. But there were times he was just a loving dad and took us to the movies or for a ride in his convertible with the top down.

If you ever needed him for something, he would always be there, like the time my car broke down at college and he came in the pouring rain at midnight to get me. He made mistakes and, while neither parent was perfect, they loved each other. My mother accepted and loved all of him. No matter what, they stood by each other and stayed together. I guess that is where I learned to tolerate a lot for the sake of love and family and to turn a blind eye to any misgivings.

Too Late

A year after Lauren was finished with chemo, my youngest sister, Cathy, called me at work.

"Lisa, Dad is on the way to the hospital, he had a heart attack. You should get here right away."

I sat at my desk a little bit in shock thinking he'd probably just need a bypass surgery or something and would be fine. No matter, I called my husband and asked him to pick the kids up from daycare and ran out the door.

When I got to the hospital and saw my five siblings and my mother sobbing, I knew I wasn't in time to say good-bye. Cathy came over to me and explained that my brother, Eddie, (named after our father) had performed CPR until the paramedics got to the house to no avail.

"He was gone before he got here. We didn't want you to know until you arrived so you wouldn't be driving upset," Cathy added.

We stayed there by his side as long as we could, each taking a turn to say our surreal good-byes. It was finally time to go. We left in disbelief of what had just happened. I asked my mom if I could take her home.

"Do you have any plans for the funeral?" I asked.

"He was only sixty-three! We never thought about it!" she said.

We passed a funeral home by our church and I asked if she wanted to stop in.

"It might be good to ask questions to at least get an idea of what needs to happen from here," I said.

My mother agreed and we went inside. We ended up making all the arrangements right then. In crisis situations, I tend to do what's needed and collapse later. My mom was relieved we got this done.

At the wake, Lauren walked up to my dad, pulling her grandmother along with her.

"Grandma, if I give Grandpa a kiss on the check, will he wake up?"

"No, sweetheart, Grandpa is with the angels now. We won't see him again until we are in heaven. But you can still feel his love in your heart." My mom, with tears rolling down her face, hugged Lauren, touched that she thought she could wake my dad up.

I Will Remember You

When Lauren got home, she went to her room and wrote something in her scribbly little handwriting. Since she had lost some of her vision, she wrote extra big and used a purple marker. I went into her room to check on her and was surprised to see what my five year old had written to her Grandpa. My mom has kept this all these years.

"I will remember you. I love you. I will be there for you. My tears run to the ground. Why did you have to die? I will forever love you. At least I'll see you when I die in heaven. It will be all for you. My

tears run down my face. I will be there for you. You are in my heart and I'll send you my love. Why did you have to die?"

Germany

With the passing of my dad, we reconnected with some family members in Germany. Upon hearing about Lauren's condition of NF1, my dad's cousin, Wilhelm Kaltenstadler, reached out to me via email. He said he knew holistic practitioners in Germany and Austria that we might want to meet and take Lauren to see. He invited the entire family to come stay with him.

That summer my mom, older sister Marion, and her daughter, Jessica, accompanied us to Germany. It was an exciting trip that started with a day layover in Paris. Chris climbed the Eiffel tower as Lauren and I walked around the beautiful grounds. We got to have lunch in a Parisian café, take a city tour, walk along the River Siene and go to a carnival. It was an amazing prelude to our trip to Munich.

Wilhelm greeted us at the airport and was so welcoming. During our stay, he took us to visit the house where my great grandparents lived and raised their fifteen children. I could feel my dad's spirit with us. I was so grateful for the opportunity to visit the country where my dad's parents were born and for the visits with the holistic doctors that Wilhelm arranged.

The first practitioner we met was a professor in Munich who ran a cancer research and retreat center that was focused on nutrition. He recommended an organic raw diet for Lauren along with some supplements. The other doctor was a friend of Wilhelm's and came from Austria to see Lauren. He performed what I can only describe as acupuncture on the tips of her fingers. She hated it so much it stuck in her mind for years!

"That was the trip where that man hurt my fingers," she would always recall.

Both specialists said Lauren's immune system was impaired from the chemo and felt their treatments would help restore her health. New ideas were continuously presented that we could not ignore. We had no way of knowing which one, if any, could possibly be "The One" to assist my baby girl.

Chris and Lauren may have only been seven and five, but they both have fond memories of this trip to Europe. Wilhelm and his family were gracious hosts. They gave us the opportunity to see so much of Germany, meet relatives we never knew we had and of course visit with cutting edge holistic doctors! It was a trip of a lifetime that my dad would have loved.

CHAPTER

Six

New Direction

Back home, we applied what we learned on our trip to Germany. This complemented what we learned from our studies of Pranic Healing – how to use *ki* (life force energy) to assist in healing. We had been taking Lauren for Pranic energy healings with an MD who was a certified Pranic Healer in New Jersey in hopes it would shrink the tumor and boost her immune system.

Lauren's positivity and faith grew and expanded but I wasn't sure if she said and did things to make me happy or because she truly felt a connection. I believe it was a combination of my influence and faith-filled experiences along with the experiences she had of her own. She genuinely seemed connected to spirit. We said prayers at dinner and Lauren liked to take the lead on this. She would always start with "Dear God, Jesus and all the angels...." Her father and brother would sometimes mock her, but faith was very important to me and Lauren, so we didn't care when they did this. When they or anyone said things she didn't want to hear, she would hold her arm out with her hand up and say, "Talk to the hand" with her girlish grin.

Remove Limiting Thoughts

Later that year, I was planning to go to the Wealth Mindset (WM) introductory workshop being offered in California with the two free tickets I had taken. My husband was not interested in coming with me, so I asked my sister Annalise. When she had to back out at the last minute, my husband reluctantly agreed that if I had no one else, he would come. It would be a decision that would change our lives forever.

During the three-day seminar, the leader reviewed techniques he used to remove limiting thoughts, beliefs and feelings that keep you from all you deserve and desire. There was a big focus on mindset: how our thoughts create our feelings and result in our actions. It was more confirmation for me about how our mind, body and spirit are all connected, and I was interested in everything this man had to say.

Whose Program Is It?

The program leader spoke of many different personal growth boot camps his company offered to help people grow and expand in all aspects of their lives and careers. My husband was a convert. From someone who didn't even want to go on the trip with me, it was a complete turn-around. He was enamored by this man and loved everything he had to offer.

They offered multiple packages during the weekend, but when they pitched the final bundled "quantum" package of all the workshops at an equally "quantum" price, my husband turned to me.

"This program is exactly what I need to take my practice to the next level."

"It sounds great, hun, and I'd love to take all these courses too. But we really can't afford it," I replied.

He insisted that it would pay for itself over time and by purchasing the big program, we got some extra perks including a trip to the Caribbean. Plus, I would be able to go to one of the workshops for free. He was so excited and persistent, and we had to make a quick decision, so I hesitantly agreed. We put it on a credit card. We'd figure out how to pay for it later.

Suddenly it was my husband's program and not mine. A few months later he went to his first workshop. The focus was on discovering your true calling and identifying your personal mission and vision for success. He came home so excited and passionate, calling himself "soaring eagle." I wish I could have been there myself.

In later reflection, I wondered if this is when he started going off in an entirely different direction.

Warrior Within

Six months later, I had a chance to go to my free workshop with my husband in beautiful western Canada. I choose the program called "Warrior" because it was all about breaking through your personal limitations: physically, mentally and spiritually. I saw a side of myself and my husband, I didn't know existed. The days were filled with many activities all intended for personal growth and enlightenment.

One exercise was particularly challenging and nerve-wracking. We were doing a high rope challenge and found ourselves thirty feet up on a platform. We had to step off together onto two parallel ropes. We pushed against each other's hands for balance. As we moved slowly across the ropes, they got farther and farther apart until we were almost a body's length from each other. We really had to look at and listen to each other or we would fall. I never liked heights and was scared, but my husband stayed calm and talked me through it and we made it to the other side. I was impressed and trusted him in a way I never had before.

As part of this workshop, we had to break into "tribes." My husband decided he wanted to be in a separate tribe from me. I would have preferred to stay together, but respected his decision. The tribes competed and during one event we literally had to climb a mountain. The task was to get your tribe members up to the peak and back down by a certain time. There were checkpoints along the way, and you got points for every team member who made it to the top and back down. The tribe with the most points was honored at dinner that night.

My husband and I started the hike together, but when I slowed down, he decided to go on without me and get to the top. I paired up with a person moving at my pace and we encouraged each other as the climb got steeper and more strenuous. When we got toward the very top, there was my husband assisting and encouraging others who were almost there. I wasn't really happy that he had left me behind, but seeing him helping others reach the top of the mountain made me proud of him. It was easier to climb back down but everyone was exhausted at this point. As I approached the finish line, there again were others who had already made it down cheering everyone on. We were taught to run not walk through the finish line and with everyone cheering, I found the strength to start running and felt exhilarated as I crossed the finish line.

One of the last activities was to walk across thirty feet of hot coals. It was incredible to me that this could be done without burning your feet. I watched closely as they demonstrated this. Then I watched person after person walk across, which gave me the courage to do the same. It was incredible! Leaving camp, I felt the same peace and connection to spirit as I had at Grand Canyon. Only this time I felt more connected to my husband than I had in a long time.

It was after this course that I found myself teaching Chris and Lauren even more how important it is to have positive intentions. There were phrases and philosophies used at the camp that were ingrained in me to this very day:

"What you focus on grows."

"How you do anything, is how you do everything."

"When emotions are high, intelligence is low."

"Run, don't walk through the finish line."

We were taught to be "warriors" in life and there is a time to be the peaceful warrior and use calm energy and a time to suck it up and charge head on. It's here that I really understood that our thoughts lead to our feelings, which influence our actions and impacts our results. I learned that I am in charge of my thoughts and what I think and believe IS my reality. I also learned it's ultimately my choice how to respond to anything that happens to me.

I felt so inspired after taking this week-long camp. It seemed like the universe had our back and was moving us to find one thing after another that helped improve our life and our mindset as we went through challenges as a family.

CHAPTER

Seven

Second Time Around

My husband was doing well in his chiropractic practice and things did seem to soar for a bit. He attributed the success to the WM courses he was taking and enjoying so much. I was also doing well and at the height of my career as director of my company's national executive briefing centers. Things were going great for us and then came more exciting news.

Dream Home

"You know that beautiful Victorian you have always loved over by the kids school?" my husband asked excitedly. "It has a big FOR SALE BY OWNER sign out front."

"Are you serious?" I could already see myself planting flowers in the yard with Lauren and sipping coffee on the front porch watching Chris play basketball.

I remembered talking to one of Lauren's daycare teachers about the house the year before. I was surprised when she told me that it was her parents' house, and they might be selling in a year or so. She gave me her number and I pinned it on the kitchen's bulletin board and forgot all about it. I couldn't believe I found it right where I put it, under a bunch of other things.

"How soon can we see the place?" I asked the man who answered the phone.

"As soon as I put my pants on!" I laughed and went to tell the kids.

Christopher was not happy. He was eight years old now and head strong. He marched up and down the hall saying, "No way, no how! I'm not moving!" Nothing I said could convince him. His best friend, Nick, lived next door and he did NOT want to move.

We took the two-minute drive to the sprawling blue Victorian with a wrap-around porch. As we walked through the house, we kept looking at each other, trying to keep our cool. The house had everything we dreamed of and more. For years we made it a New Year's Eve tradition to write down the things we want to create for the coming year. We would put our lists in a silver box on the mantle. This house had everything on our list, right down to the in-ground pool, huge master bedroom and fireplace. It was almost too incredible to be true, as if we'd manifested this perfect home exactly as we envisioned it.

While we were touring the interior, Chris was outside and met the neighbors – two boys from his afterschool program. Now he was excited!

"Mom, work your magic!" he said when he came inside to choose which bedroom would be his. Lauren followed suit and asked, "Which bedroom will be yours mommy?" Then pointed to the room right next to the master and said, "I want this one so I can be right next to you."

We made an offer on the house that day and incredibly sold our house in two weeks' time. We were in the house before the kids started school in the fall. It felt as if it was meant to be. Now we had our dream home, complete with a white picket – well, PVC – fence. Our family was happy and seemingly healthy. We even got a dog, Jasper, a small black cockapoo with a white neck that Lauren said made him look like a tuxedo. We were living the American dream.

Someone to Help Me See

Our new house didn't need anything major except for some painting. George, our go-to painter always called my husband Doc. Over the years, we became friendly with him and his wife, Maritza. They were spending a lot of time painting our new home and re-staining the deck on our wrap-around porch. Maritza and I talked about our daughters. She was always kind and compassionate regarding Lauren, and I appreciated having her to chat with.

Lauren went to the ophthalmologist every three months since her chemo stopped. Though she never complained about her vision getting worse, the eye doctor confirmed the vision in her right eye was progressively declining. It was down in June, got a little worse in September but the doctors weren't alarmed until January of 2005. That's when the results of the next routine MRI showed the tumor looked enlarged. The doctors felt with the progression of vision loss and growth of the tumor, it was time for another round of chemo. They recommended the same protocol as before. Lauren was six years old, four years since her first treatment. So much for the American dream.

There was no denying the decrease in her vision, but the doctors weren't sure if the tumor had grown or if it had just changed shape because of the surrounding fluid in her brain. My heart sank with the news of having to restart chemo right away. On top of that, they told us she should be evaluated for another type of therapy called orientation and mobility, or O&M, to help her navigate at school and home in case her vision continued to worsen.

When we got home from the doctor, George and Maritza were at the house and just packing up from a day of work on the deck. Maritza took one look at me.

"Is everything okay?" I shook my head no and she held me as I wept.

I pulled it together and Maritza got in the car with George. I thought they'd left but I heard a knock on the door. It was George and what he said confused me.

"Maritza felt something while you embraced," he said. "She didn't know if you'd be open to hearing it."

I consider myself a Type A, rational, no-nonsense businesswoman. I am very down to earth and practical. I appreciate logic, systems and organization. Faith was taught in my Catholic upbringing, but metaphysics and spiritual realms were really not in my repertoire. I had studied and practiced meditation, and even utilized the services of some energy healers, but this would be a completely new area I was about to dive into, and this is when my spiritual journey began in earnest.

I walked over to Maritza to hear what she had to say. She told me about her gifts of sight and healing and how she felt drawn to assist me and Lauren. From that day forward she has been right there by my side sharing faith, comforting words and compassion. She would become my spiritual mentor and best friend – a true miracle who showed up in Divine timing, right when I needed her. Over the years I would come to rely on her insight more and more.

Maritza and I would explore the world of spirit and metaphysics in a way I still struggle to explain. We talked about how important it is to have faith and she shared scriptures with me that had helped her through tough times. After talking to her, I decided to go back to church for a sense of community. Most important of all, I began my slow awakening to the understanding that everything is vibration and we are essentially energetic, spiritual beings having a physical experience.

Different Reaction

Things were not going well during Lauren's second round of chemo. Though it was the same exact protocol as the first chemo, she was having a completely different reaction to it. Lauren was throwing up, having fevers and was neutropenic (low white blood cell count) for the first time. I tried to tell myself this was a natural way for the body to react and release toxins, but she was struggling, and I was feeling emotionally wiped out.

Somehow, we got Lauren through two months of chemo and went in for a follow-up eye exam. That's when things got even worse. Lauren's vision in her right eye declined further to 20/200 and her eye doctor told us she was now legally blind. I almost couldn't bear to stay in the room while he was telling us. My head spun with news we never expected to hear, especially with all we were doing both with chemo and holistically.

The next step was to have an emergency MRI and see if the tumor was growing. We immediately got in touch with her local oncologist as well as the top specialist in DC.

The good news was the MRI showed no visible growth of the tumor, but the bad news was the chemo was evidently not working since her vision was getting worse.

"She is too young for radiation," the specialist in DC said. I hadn't even considered radiation an option. He recommended we stick with the current chemo until the end of the induction period and watch if her vision and tumor stabilize. He said if the tumor or vision worsens, we could try two other chemo drugs. We followed up with our local pediatric oncologist and he concurred. We researched the other chemotherapies and decided they were not good options because they had many side effects.

Things were moving so fast now and not in a good way. I didn't feel like I had time to react; I just did whatever needed to be done. In less than ten days, we went from routine chemo visits to meeting with a man from the Commission for the Blind who told me about the devices and services Lauren would need for her low vision. I was scheduling follow-up appointments practically daily, handling the family and doing my best at work.

One day while my husband was away, Lauren came down with a fever of 105.1. I put her in the tub in an attempt to cool down the fever, gave her Tylenol and called my husband. He called the hospital and they said to bring her right over. They prescribed three days of antibiotics. I sat down to collect myself when I got back home.

I was emotionally shot at this point and beside myself. Between all the Pranic Healings, prayer, nutrition, chemo and spiritual support Lauren was getting, I hoped and even expected that things would improve. Instead, her vision was worse, and I was constantly watching her for new symptoms. Now she had a scary-high fever out of the blue. I was home alone with two kids to take care of and feeling defeated. If there is spiritual support all around us all the time like Maritza said, I could sure use some now.

Emperor's New Clothes

We kept looking for the treatment that would do the trick and heal our daughter. My husband was away attending a chiropractic seminar. While there, he learned about a technique called "muscle testing" which is used to determine where the body is deficient in nutrients. He met another chiropractor, Dr. V, that developed a system of using a combination of muscle testing and magnetic therapy. He said he had great results with his patients, some who were high profile. We were impressed and hopeful his system could do the same for Lauren. My husband would take Lauren to Dr. V's office on Long Island, where we lived, and also to his office in Florida so she wouldn't miss any sessions.

During this time, I was reading many books. I read *"Hands of Light"* by Barbara Brennan which made a huge impact on me. She built a school of healing, now located in Florida, which trains people on her healing techniques. I found a local practitioner and started taking Lauren to see her. I continued to read about various energy and healing approaches. Over time I would become certified in a number of modalities myself, including becoming a Reiki Master and hypnotherapist. But I am getting ahead of myself.

At this point in time, we were just being exposed to many alternative healing techniques. There were times I wondered if I was buying into the Emperor's New Clothes, letting myself be convinced of something I really couldn't see. The muscle testing, magnetic therapy and energy healings were all so intangible. But it didn't prevent me from pursuing them. They gave me hope. The people who practiced them were so well meaning and believed so strongly in what they practiced, and these techniques were also so gentle compared to the harsh chemo. I tied back our philosophy: if it couldn't hurt her and might help her, why not try it?

Then, one night I was sleeping beside Lauren who wanted me with her when she felt so sick. She woke me up shortly after midnight.

"Mommy, I have to tell you about the angel that just came to visit!" Lauren said.

She'd been telling me about dreams of angels for a while. When I opened my eyes to look at her, I saw tiny circles of white lights over Lauren. At first, I was scared but then I felt a sense of peace and calm. I got up to wake my husband but as soon as I did, they disappeared.

I could swear I was awake, but in the morning I wondered if it was all a dream.

The more I learned about holistic healing and spirituality, and the more I meditated, the more dreams I was having. I also started seeing spiritual images in the sky and elsewhere in nature. It was all comforting and I felt like it meant miracles were possible even though chemo was making her sick, and things didn't seem like they were improving.

Both Chris and Lauren were seeing signs too. On the way home from work one day, Chris pointed up at some come clouds in the sky and said, "Look Mommy, a cross!" I looked up and saw a very clear cross in the clouds. I was so ready for a miracle, and I guess so was he. We were hoping signs like this promised good things to come.

I helped Lauren do her affirmations every day. She continued with her standard, "I am healthy, I am strong," but also added some additional statements. "I have the power in my body to heal itself so all my healthy cells get to work right now and give the unhealthy cells food from my angels – so they can be healthy again!"

She drew a picture and explained it to me. "There are cells that had three, then six, then a hundred and fifty healthy cells where they used to be unhealthy ones!"

Another Shoe Drops

We took Lauren for another eye exam four weeks after her last one to check her vision. It dropped again from 20/200 to 8/200. It didn't come as a total surprise to me because I had noticed her moving closer and closer to the T.V. to watch her favorite programs.

She was also putting her face really close to the paper when reading or writing. I thought we were going to at least finish chemo, but both of her oncologists in New York and DC agreed we should stop this treatment and consider other options.

She had just turned seven years old and had been through two rounds of chemo and was considered legally blind. It would be four more weeks before she could start any other kind of treatment. Her little body needed to rest and recover. Our local doctor said to come back in two weeks so he could do bloodwork and discuss options with us. It was hard for me to get my head wrapped around all of this.

Stop Treatment

My heart sank. I cried for days and felt like I was having a mini-meltdown. It was decision time. The doctor's offered other chemo options that would be much harsher on her body. The other option was to stop and use a wait-and-see approach. After much discussion and tears, my husband and I decided to not pursue other chemo treatments at this time. Lauren's doctors were not one hundred percent on board but agreed watching and waiting was a reasonable choice.

What got me through the night at this point was knowing that we, and so many other people, were doing all they could – doctors, therapists, holistic practitioners, and of course, our friends and families with their prayers and just being there. I was like a sponge, taking classes and studying whatever I could on health and healing of body, mind and spirit. If there was something out there that could help Lauren, I was going to find it. I not only learned about hands-on healing, but also about distance healing and how we all have the ability to send light and love through both of these methods. Healers would explain how they were merely the vehicle being used to send energy in the form of unconditional love. It pours through them from "Source" or "God."

The connection between the body, mind and spirit was now undeniable to me. I had even felt energy in my hands during various trainings and healing sessions. From what I read and experienced, I knew the physical experience is not all we have. This is a concept that was also discussed and experienced during the Warrior camp I had been to. It had a profound effect on me. I remember a moment by the waterside early one morning when a thought occurred to me. "It is only in stillness that we can see our true reflection." It was time for us to be still.

These concepts remained very important to me and would continue to impact me in the days, months and years that lie ahead. It's the story we tell ourselves about what's happening that is real, I remembered. That's why two people in the same exact situation can walk away with two very different experiences.

I would always remember that we may not have control over all the situations in our life, but we do have control over how we react. I would then ask myself: "What story is it that I want to tell?" When it came to Lauren, the story I wanted to tell was one of a miracle. I wanted it to be about a little girl who had a family who loved her so much and had so much faith that she got the miracle of health and well-being and her sight restored. How could she not with all that we were doing?

CHAPTER

Eight

Light And Love

I kept my strength and hopes up that things would get better for Lauren. Though chemo stopped, we continued with the other holistic treatments and healings. Magnetic therapy was one of those things we continued with. The technique was simple: we placed several blocks on and around her body while she was laying down. It was supposed to have a healing effect. She was always so great about doing whatever crazy thing mom or dad wanted to try. I used these occasions of lying in bed with her to talk about our day or read to her and of course let her know how much I love her.

See Beyond

"I already did my affirmations," Lauren said. "Would you read *Clifford* while I close my eyes so I can see if I can remember what the pictures look like?"

"Lauren, are you ever afraid of losing your vision?" I asked.

"No, mommy. I actually feel lucky!"

"Lucky? Why?" I asked.

"Because some other children never had their vision, but I know what it's like to see. I remember everything – the flowers, the trees, the butterflies...and your beautiful face."

Tears welled in my eyes. Maybe having physical vision wasn't the most important thing for Lauren, but I never gave up hope she could have that miracle. Yes, this child could already see with her heart and maybe seeing with the eyes of the body isn't what she is here to do. As a mother, though, I was still not ready to give up hope.

"You're amazing," I told her.

"Why am I amazing?" she asked, giggling.

"Because you just are!" I kissed her all over her face and told her all the reasons why I loved her (as I often did) and how much the whole family loved her too.

"I know they love me Mommy! And God and Jesus and all the angels do, too."

"Of course they do," I said, "We all do!"

Lauren spoke of angels often and I knew she had all the angels from above and all the angels here on earth surrounding her. Our family on both sides had come to visit over the weekend. We all cushioned Lauren with love. It had meant so much to have them close, and to know they'd be there, strong, loving and ready to see us through whatever may come.

Even with all this support, the tension of waiting, intending and hoping was wearing on me. I worked hard on trusting that the outcome of all Lauren's medical and spiritual treatments would be for the highest good, but sometimes I doubted. If I could only believe enough or find the right practice or unblock whatever was in her way, Lauren's sight could be restored, and she could experience perfect health. I went back and forth between feeling that everything was as it should be and that something had to improve. I was ready for breakthroughs and solutions.

Energy healers were focused on sending Lauren light and love and doing either hands-on or remote healing with her. One of them suggested I talk to her about forgiveness, so I added it to Lauren's daily affirmations and told her how important it is to love and forgive ourselves. Another healer suggested I stop talking to Lauren so much about her health and healing. Was I confusing her? Or filling her up with too much false hope and expectation?

Most of the healers were also intuitive, which meant they received messages from spirit and would share them with me. One said Lauren was a very evolved being.

"You and your daughter will be a light in this world and Lauren will see beyond her eyes," another said. I wasn't sure exactly what that meant but already knew this child saw with her heart as well as her eyes.

No Limits

My friend and co-worker, Lisa, knew this well and felt Lauren was heaven sent. She recalls the very first time she met Lauren. It was back when she attended daycare at my company, during one of the many times I would bring her to my desk after having lunch in the company cafeteria. Lisa had her head down, busy with work and she looked up to see this little girl with her hand out, holding a candy.

"Would you like a Werther?" she asked. Then Lauren would start with her questions:

"Do you have a husband and children?" she asked.

"I just got married," Lisa told Lauren.

"Well, be sure he treats you like a princess," Lauren said.

She ended their conversation by asking Lisa if she could give her a hug, which touched her heart. Lisa and I would become very close friends over the years. As our relationship grew, so did her relationship with Lauren.

Lisa said anytime she was around Lauren, it would lift her spirits and they'd always be smiling or laughing together. Lauren had a way of taking her mind away from wherever it was and filled her heart with joy. She and my other co-workers always looked forward to her visits and the gifts she would bring whether it was a Werther's candy, a picture made out of foamies (foam cut-outs in all different shapes that we got from the arts and crafts store) or just a hug. Lisa kept a note Lauren wrote her that had foamies on it with pink and purple hearts.

"Dear Lisa, I love you, I miss you and hope you have a fantastic day. Love, Lauren."

As Lauren began to lose her vision, she needed a little help to write her name so it would be big and a little scribbly. Lisa said every time she looked at the picture with her scribbly name, it reminded her of this little girl with no limits.

Lisa would later experience some very tough times of her own. She says she never forgot Lauren's courage and positivity which helped her get through her darkest days when she lost her infant twins. Lauren's kind words and bravery was always an inspiration to Lisa, especially during this otherwise unbearable time.

Lauren would always tell her everything was going to be ok and somehow that gave her the strength to get through. When Lisa got pregnant again, she started to get really scared as she approached delivery, thinking about the loss of her two little ones. She said Lauren helped take away her fears by sharing her loving words and reassuring her once again that everything was going to be ok. The fact that Lauren was able to endure all she did and stay positive and happy was what gave Lisa her added strength.

"It may sound simple, but it had a profound effect on me," Lisa said.

"To this day, I think of Lauren as my Go-To Girl for strength, courage, bravery and compassion. She was a true beacon of love and light."

Little Miracles

I often wondered how many miracles you need to have in order to believe in miracles. I tried to pay attention to small miracles that came our way. Lauren did seem to have a way to brighten everyone's day, including my own. People were always attracted to her. I remember one day Lauren and I went to the eyeglass store and chatted with two ladies there. After speaking with Lauren and hearing a little about her story, each said they had something special they wanted to give her. One gave her rose petal oil from St. Francis of Assisi and the other gave her Holy Water from our Lady of Lourdes in France. I was not about to say no to anything and thanked them for their gifts.

It had snowed earlier that day and when we got home, I decided to make a snowman with the kids. We were getting cold, so I just threw a few more shovels of snow at the snowman and went inside.

"That was a really cool angel you made out of the snow," my husband said when he got home.

"I didn't make an angel," I said.

He took me outside and showed me that there were two very clear wings and arms that were folded over the snowman, as well as hands that made it look like it was praying. I felt like we had signs of hope, love and kindness all around us and our decision to discontinue chemo seemed like the right one. Yes, I had to multitask to keep up with all of Lauren's needs for her low vision in our home and at school with her teachers, therapists and other daily activities. In addition, there was caring for Christopher, his activities and handling my responsibilities at work. But it was just what I had to deal with. Every family has its challenges. This was ours.

Handling It

My husband was taking two or three courses a year with WM and he was gone for a week at a time. He also traveled for his chiropractic practice to attend seminars, and when he did, it put a lot of pressure on me. I did want him to go and have transformational experiences.

However, I also felt like he was getting two or three vacations a year while I was back home holding down the fort. It felt unfair.

He kept telling me how these courses were going to change our lives. I wasn't really seeing the return on the investment, and I said so. He got a little offended.

"It takes time," he said.

I would have loved to take these self-growth classes myself but there wasn't the time or the money. Plus, his travels always came at extremely inconvenient times. I was handling it, but it would have been a lot easier if I had my husband home with me. Oddly, Lauren also seemed to get sick every time he went away – anything from running a fever to needing to go to the hospital. It was challenging enough to manage everything going on with him home. It was more difficult when he was gone. It's hard to see the light when you feel frustrated and alone.

Getting It Right

On top of everything, the magnetic therapy didn't seem to be working. My frustration was boiling over. Dr. V kept telling us things *would* improve. Even though my husband was usually the one to talk with Dr. V, I called him myself, demanding answers. I needed to see results or confirm if we were doing it right.

"You can't do it wrong, it just takes time" he told me.

The tension left my body. Maybe this would just take more time. Perhaps I needed to be more patient. I had been working so hard, trying so many things, doing my best to hold it all together. Fighting for everything was such a battle. I thought if only I could get it right, we could heal Lauren. I decided to keep giving Lauren the supplements he prescribed and continue the magnetic therapy. I'd also go with her to the doctor visits to ask any additional questions I had. I felt better after the call.

It may sound like I was conflicted between looking for miraculous healings and thinking my daughter just had small issues we had to deal with as they came up. The truth is I didn't think of Lauren as sick but did understand these were serious issues we had to address. It was the same rationale we used if Christopher needed braces or a cast for a broken arm. To be fair, that is how the doctors put it. Tackle the next thing, keep moving forward, keep things normal. Expect her to have a long, productive life. Never did they ever say or suggest that this thing could take her life. Nor could I ever imagine a world without her light shining in it.

You're Such a B-

Chris was involved with Boy Scouts and a lot of sports. With my husband's late work schedule and his traveling, I often relied on other parents to pick him up and drop him off at home between my working and taking care of Lauren. I thought these parents understood our situation and didn't mind helping out because we lived so close. Then, one weekend Chris told me he wasn't going to the birthday party of one of his closest friends. It was a sleepover in Montauk which was a few hours away.

"There isn't room for me in the car," he said.

I was taken aback and called a couple of the moms to ask about it, and that's when they let me have it.

"You are such a 'B,'" one of them said to me. "You're not the only mom who works full-time," she added.

Apparently, they'd resented me for some time for not doing my fair share of carpooling. The other woman told me I was "the invisible mom," and that other working parents made it to the soccer practices and games to show up for their sons. It touched a very deep part of my heart and soul and pained me. In that moment I questioned if I was truly being there enough for Chris. I was hurt, too, because they'd never asked me what was going on at home or ever thought to ask me to come over for a cup of coffee so they could find out. I really would have appreciated that every now and again. They knew Lauren had a lot going on, but it didn't seem to matter. I was doing my best to be there as much as I could for my son and my daughter. How could they not understand or see that, I thought to myself.

I always said that Lauren's situation brought out the best or worst in people. I've learned that Maya Angelou was right: When someone shows you who they are, believe them the first time. This would not be the only instance when I would need to apply this philosophy. From then on, I resolved that I'd keep doing my best to be there for both my children and I would not rely on those parents anymore. Sometimes you have to be your own light.

Media Magnet

I found out about a horseback riding program at a nearby stable that specialized in therapeutic riding. Lauren started lessons which were great in so many ways. They had an instructor who worked with visually impaired children and used "sidewalkers" (volunteers) to call out letters so the rider knew which direction to steer the horse. It was great exercise and Lauren loved the independence of being able to ride and direct a horse. Even better were the sidewalkers: all teenage girls. She could gab away while riding and make new friends.

Wherever we went, people, and even the media, were attracted to Lauren. She seemed to be a media magnet. A local news station was doing a feature on the therapeutic riding program. Lauren was interviewed during her lesson. She was on television and in the newspaper. From there, she was interviewed many more times by other media and news stations. Once on a ski trip hosted by STRIDE (Sports and Therapeutic Recreation Instruction/Development Education), Lauren participated in an event for the visually impaired and won a medal. Sure enough, she was interviewed by the local TV station. She was also selected to appear on the STRIDE brochure the following year using a picture from that event. All of this was so much fun for her and nice that the attention was for finishing a race, rather than finishing a round of chemo.

Hug Collector

After Lauren's next MRI, I was relieved when we got confirmation that the tumor had not changed. The news made it easier to stick with our decision of no more chemo. You would never know from her demeanor or from looking at her that her vision was impaired. She was just a sweet little girl with glasses who had such compassion for others and wanted to have fun.

While I was chatting with the nurses after the MRI, Lauren walked over to a woman who was sitting in the waiting room by herself.

"I'm a hug collector," she said and proceeded to hug the woman and talk about how she just had an MRI. When I walked over, the woman said Lauren was a little angel.

"I'm here for an MRI too," she said. "I was alone and very scared, but Lauren made me smile. If this little one can do it, so can I!"

As we walked away Lauren shouted, "Remember to sign my guest book, it's LaurensVision.com!"

My sister, Annalise, and I built the website. It was something I thought would be good for Lauren to have as a place for people she met to leave her written messages. I would read the messages to her at the end of each night, and she always looked forward to it. That night, not only did the woman sign Lauren's guestbook, but so did another woman who was watching their whole interaction.

"Lauren, you are one special little lady. You are so kind and sweet and I couldn't wait to sign your guestbook and say hi," she wrote.

Over the years, Lauren had thousands of people sign her guest book. I'm sad to say that the hosting site shut down and I ended up losing the files, but will never forget all the beautiful messages people wrote!

Suck It Up Princess

I set up meetings with Lauren's teachers and therapists to refocus on school and be sure that Lauren was keeping up with her peers. She now had an aide at school, but I wanted her to have as much independence as she could and not be excluded from experiences like going outdoors for recess. I wanted her to be given the same opportunities as the other kids, and I advocated that she be encouraged to push herself, take care of herself, and speak up for herself, too. I was adamant that she was going to be involved in everything she normally would and socialize as any girl her age would want to. I required that she never be excluded from anything.

If there was something she didn't want to do (mostly schoolwork), we'd joke with her and say, "Suck it up, Princess." And we were right there with her, sucking it up too. We set a high bar for her and the life she could have. I was showing her how to live a high-quality life no matter what. She always knew that her Mommy had her back. I guess you could say I was teaching her how to be my little warrior princess and teaching her when to use her calm energy and when to put on her armor as I had learned to get through life's trials and tribulations.

Miraculous News

Lauren was getting MRIs and eye check-ups monthly since we stopped her chemo in February 2005. Every MRI showed no change. In June, we finally got amazing news. Her eye doctor said the vision in her right eye had improved and he didn't know how to explain it. He wanted to know more about the other treatments we were doing. We were thrilled and so very, very thankful. Exactly what made the difference? Which treatment or practice? Where should I double down on my efforts? I would affirm, "Lauren's path is in God's hands, and I am here to serve and assist in whatever way I can." Sometimes you have to let go and let God.

With things improving, Lauren had another surgery in December. This time it was to remove her mediport! She once again impressed the medical staff with her courage through this procedure. The beginning of 2006 felt like things were coming together. What others might call a challenging life felt pretty miraculous for us. When Lauren was stable, life for all of us was stable. Chris was now nine and Lauren was seven. Both of them were happy, had plenty of friends and were doing well in school. They participated in many activities like dance, sports, piano and horseback riding. Life felt normal. I was joyful in these simple things and everything that was unfolding and felt like the worst was behind us.

My husband held his first workshop at his chiropractic office on Total Wellness and I led an introduction to meditation segment. Teaching meditation felt so rewarding. It was at this time I felt something deep inside telling me to write about Lauren and our journey as a family. I always knew in my heart there is a higher good at work here and wanted to share it with others. I reflected on the message given during a healing that my daughter and I would be a light for the world. What might that look like? I wondered.

One day, Lauren declared, "Today, I get my vision back!"

"How would you feel about that?" I asked.

"Mommy, I'm just glad to be alive! I am happy and I know God made me the way he thought was best!" She was always so positive and happy. She changed up her affirmations to include her having her sight back and shouted them out loud.

I was also realizing that while I thought I was here to love and serve Lauren, she was here to love me and show me how to live in a way I never imagined. One way she did that was by teaching me we can love life even if it isn't picture perfect. I couldn't be more of a testament to the saying that "Life is what happens when your plans don't work out." Lauren wasn't concerned about plans – a far cry from how I am. She just enjoyed her life, and I renewed my commitment to help her live her best possible life.

Did I wish that my daughter was perfectly healthy? Yes, of course I did. But could I also celebrate this life she shared with me no matter what? Yes, but I still hoped (and expected) a miracle: perfect health was possible for her.

Section Two
ENERGY

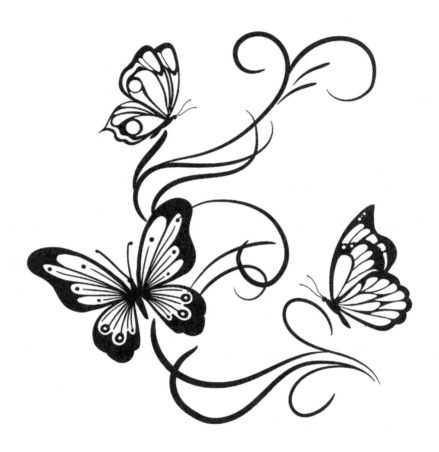

CHAPTER

Nine

Karmic Connections

Three months after we removed Lauren's mediport, she had another eye exam. She had just turned eight and was in second grade. This time the doc felt her vision had declined further and recommended she start to learn Braille. Her vision teacher at school, however, read the report and based on his interpretation and observation of Lauren, felt her functional vision had remained the same. My emotions would always swing whenever there was a shift in what things meant for Lauren's life. I relied on my faith to keep a positive attitude, but it would take a long time before I learned that staying in faith meant that crappy things, and even things that bring great sorrow, could still come my way. Even faith didn't guarantee there would be no pain.

It was easy to feel good when everything seemed ok. Life was such a roller coaster of emotions with Lauren's health swinging from one direction to another. I did affirmations along with Lauren and declared, "I am abundance and well-being," but I didn't feel it. I believed in karma and that if you are a good person, good things will come to you. I wanted to hear my inner guidance confirm that, but when I meditated, I questioned what I heard. I was beat down by the news Lauren should start Braille and feared for her future.

Newfound Friend

Over the years, fear and uncertainty had become unwelcome friends. I could see them coming and feel my body shift into anxiety at their arrival. It was time for me to look fear in the face. As if the Universe heard I needed support, I came across books that talked about fear in a unique ways. One explained that fear is False Evidence Appearing Real. The other said FEAR is a gift from our Creator to assist us, not destroy us. It went on to explain that fear is feedback designed to help us take proper action: fight or flight response. Based on whatever Frightening Event we experience, we need to Ask ourselves: What is an appropriate Reaction to the event?

It then hit me that it all comes back to changing our thoughts and focusing on the positive to motivate us to take actions that allow us to achieve the results we desire. Whenever fear showed up, I would always try to ask myself, "What can I do to MOVE from this place of fear toward the place I want to be?" I asked it more times than I care to count.

Trip to Philly

I re-grounded myself in positive thoughts and got back to the task of finding ways to assist Lauren. I kept reading books like *Getting in the Gap* by Wayne Dyer and *Co-creating at Its Best*, co-written by Esther Hicks. Then I came across a book by Michael Bradford called *The Healing Energy of Your Hands*. In it, he spoke about the hands-on healing techniques he learned and practiced. His contact information was in the back of the book, so I decided to reach out to him.

Bradford said he was going to be spending time in Philadelphia to work on his next book. He was moved by Lauren's journey and felt like he could assist her. He said he would be happy to meet with us while there. I decided to take her to see him. As soon as we arrived, he spoke with Lauren for a bit and then had some interesting things to say about her past life. He said he felt that losing her vision was allowing her to play out some karma she carried with her from a past life. He explained that it had something to do with a past relationship and traumatic experience she had. He described a horse that was very special to her in that lifetime and that somehow led her soul to make some critical decisions. None of this made much sense at the time. He finally did hands-on healing work on her which was more of what I expected. I was happy I took her to see him. I never thought about karma from a past life. It made me curious, and I had to investigate.

Past Life Connection

When we got home, I asked Maritza what she thought about a karmic connection and if she felt she could connect to past lives and see if that would provide any additional insight as to what was going on with Lauren in this life. Maritza had not done anything like that before, but she agreed to try. I always asked her questions about what was possible with her intuitive abilities. Above all, she considers herself a healer, but also has the gift of sight. As she explains it, things are shown to her like a movie.

She connected to spirit to inquire. What she saw shocked us both. She described Lauren's past life as a wealthy young woman who lived during the time of World War II. She was married to an older German soldier who was responsible for a concentration camp near their home. She had no idea what was happening at the camp until one day when she rode her horse out to see her husband and was horrified by what she witnessed.

When the war ended, the German soldiers were being rounded up for arrest and prosecution. Her husband fled and abandoned her and their children. The villagers came for him and assumed he was in their home. When he didn't come out, they burned it down and she died with her two children in the fire.

Her soul was devastated and felt unworthy because of the life she lived. She also felt unloved because her husband had abandoned her and their family. She vowed to never again see the horrors of the world and wanted to be punished for living a lavish life while others had suffered at the hands of her husband. Could it be possible that Lauren was losing her vision in this lifetime because of some sort of vow or contract she made before she got here?

Our Soul Contract

Maritza and I both needed time to process this past life scenario. Even Maritza could not believe what she was being shown. Since then, I've read many books about how our souls continue on past death, including the classic by prominent psychiatrist Brian Weiss, *Many Lives, Many Masters,* and the popular *Embraced by the Light* based on the near-death experience of Betty Eadie. From them I learned that souls could play out karma in a future life and even agree to join forces and assist each other in healing on their journeys. Did I choose to come back to assist Lauren in her healing this lifetime? I wondered.

We continued our exploration and were shown that when Lauren was ready to come back to have another physical experience, she wanted to pick up where she left off – feeling defeated, unloved and unworthy. She wanted to pay her debt for all the wrongs of her past life. She essentially wanted to atone. But we were shown that the purpose of coming back is not to relive or re-pay debts or to suffer at all. The whole reason for living is to learn and grow in love.

I know this might sound crazy; it sounded crazy to me at first too. But I was searching for answers, and this seemed to make sense. I was here to show Lauren that she was loved and worthy of an incredible life. I was here to lift her spirit and let her know just how unconditionally loved she was. Lauren did not keep it all for herself. She shared unconditional love with me and everyone she met.

All of this still begged to ask additional questions? Are past lives real? Do we reincarnate to heal, resolve or put closure on things from the past? Or as some scientists or psychologists would say, is this our mind creating a story or metaphor in order to explain the unexplainable. All I knew was this gave some possible explanation for why this was all happening and something that I might be able to assist with.

Rainbow Bead Girl

As a part of her home OT exercises, Lauren made "pop-it" bead bracelets. The plastic, colorful beads were easy to pop together. She loved to make them and give them out, especially to people who she thought needed some inspiration. We started calling her "Rainbow Bead Girl." I made business cards for her with a rainbow and added this info to her website. These bracelets provided the added bonus of being a great conversation starter. She would always be sure to hand out a business card with each bracelet and tell people to be sure to sign the guest book on LaurensVision.com.

The pop-it bead bracelets were nice but they easily fell apart. So Lauren and I went to our local arts and crafts store to look for new beads. We found adorable beads in the shape of stars, butterflies and hearts that she could string together. She said they were perfect and started making them right away. Lauren was particular about the order they were in – they always had to be STAR, BUTTERFLY, HEART and one day she started saying she put LOVE, ENERGY and POWER in every bead. This became her signature gift and expression.

There was some kind of magic in these bracelets because everyone seemed to love them, the message they carried and the little girl who delivered it. I always said that Lauren may have lost her sight but never her hopes and dreams she had for her life. These bracelets became symbolic of how she lived – with love, energy and power!

The Aruba Connection

My sister, Marion, and her family had a timeshare in Aruba and went every year. One year they asked us to join them. On the plane ride over, we met a young couple that were from New Jersey. Matt was in his twenties and was warm and friendly with a great smile. Shannon was his fiancée, and they were with her family on their annual trip to Aruba. Matt sat behind Lauren, and she flirted and gabbed with him and Shannon the entire four plus hours. As we landed, we found out they were staying at the same hotel. We ended up sitting next to this family every day at the pool. Lauren captured their hearts as she told them her bad knock-knock jokes and gave away her bracelets and business cards that she made sure were packed for the trip.

It turns out we were all taking the same flight back to New York, only the flight was full and Matt was getting bumped because he had booked his trip separately. We were right behind them on the check-in line and Matt turned to us and said, "Wow, this really stinks because I have to get back to work." Lauren immediately turned to us and asked if we could give up our seats so Matt could fly back with his beautiful Shannon. My husband and I looked at each other and only took a minute to agree with our compassionate little girl. This family was so kind and good to Lauren the whole week, and we did not have to rush back to anything. Even though this meant lugging our bags around and checking back into a hotel for one night, we were happy to do it and happy to have one more night in Paradise. The airline covered our night at a hotel right on the beach and we got to have dinner while watching the sunset. It was then that we decided we would make Aruba an annual family tradition as well.

We stayed in touch with Matt and Shannon and would visit each other occasionally even though they lived a few hours away in Jersey. Matt worked for a radio station and remembered how Lauren loved the Jonas Brothers. One day he called her and asked, "How would you and Chris like to see the Jonas Brothers with me and Shannon at Jones Beach Theater?"

"O-M-G! Like, totally!" she said, sounding just like the valley girl she and Shannon pretended to be while they joked around in Aruba. They had a great time at the concert and continued to speak to Lauren often on the phone. She loved telling them more knock-knock jokes and also made sure Matt was treating Shannon like the princess she was.

"Remember to tell Shannon how beautiful, smart and magnificent she is!" Lauren reminded Matt.

They were smitten with Lauren and loved her positive energy and couldn't believe what an amazing happy soul she was despite all she had been through. They even invited Lauren to their wedding. While we couldn't go because of a last-minute surgery, the special connection they shared continued.

A New Path

It was a great summer and Lauren also got to attend Camp Helen Keller where she made new friends. She was happy distributing her bracelets to everyone she met. In the fall, my husband attended his last WM workshop on leadership. At this event, he had the opportunity to go on stage and did a presentation that poked fun at the leader of the program. He thought he may have offended him because afterward he was summoned to speak with the leader privately. But instead of being upset, the program lead was impressed with my husband's stage presence, humor and charisma and asked if he would consider becoming a trainer for their program.

We discussed it when he got home, he could barely contain his excitement. My husband loved being on stage, he felt it was his calling. "I'll do it part-time," he said. "We'll make it work." I wondered if this could be part of his karma – to help people grow and change while he helped Lauren share her story and love with the world. Whatever else this choice was about, I had no way of knowing the dramatic impact it would have on our family and our lives.

Pathways to Health

I started a new path of my own focusing on holistic approaches to well-being and became certified in different healing modalities. I did a Reiki certification so I could do healings on Lauren and myself and met with Shamans who practiced sound and energy healing. I was intrigued and curious about alternate approaches to healing, so I continued to work with herbalists and tried many other holistic approaches including Iridology, The Alexander Technique and the Grunwald Eye Body Method to name a few. Though I sometimes questioned these methods, I knew there was more than one pathway to health and well-being.

One day I met a man who told me about a training center called Pathways to Health which I couldn't believe was only ten minutes from my house. They offered traditional psychotherapy and a wide range of holistic and metaphysic courses on chakras, the spirit's journey, a healing technique called An-Ra, hypnotherapy certification and much more, including interfaith spiritual services on Sundays. After going for a short time, I knew I had found a new home.

While my husband started his new part-time gig as a motivational trainer, I took class after class at Pathways including weekly guided meditation. Pathways was the one thing I did for myself to get out of the house and center myself. Lauren and I attended the monthly spiritual service. The boys went a few times but weren't that interested. It was nice to be with a community of like-minded spiritual people. I became very friendly with the co-founders, Judith Grant and William Bezmen. I think Lauren mostly went for the donuts and cookies served after the spiritual service, but I was glad to have her with me.

My Ribbon of Truth

During Sunday service Judy would often talk about the process she uses when doing research on topics for her sermon and coined it the "ribbon of truth." She explained how she connects common strands of facts to formulate a basis of truth. What I have come to learn is that "truth" is also unique from person to person and even for an individual at different times in their life. What was true for me yesterday may not be my truth today and what is true for me today may not be my truth tomorrow. It is important to realize that our truth is not only based on facts but also based on our personal experiences.

I have been going to Pathways attending their Sunday Service and have taken every class and workshop they offer for over 10 years. I was drawn to them to learn more about faith, spirit and holistic healing methods. My truth is that there are many options to explore, both Western medicine as well as Eastern healing philosophies. I was on a constant quest of seeking what I could find and what the "ribbon of truth" was on healing a person.

Since finding Pathways, I went on to become a certified hypnotherapist, An-Ra healer and have had the opportunity to study and grow in my knowledge of energy healing and beyond.

Needless to say, Pathways became an integral part of my life and spiritual growth. I continued to be fascinated and drawn by the world of metaphysics and all it could offer Lauren as a chance to heal completely. Though Maritza already was already *awake* to her gifts of healing and intuition, she came with me to many events at Pathways because she also wanted to expand her spiritual knowledge and growth. She was my friend through all our family's struggles, but what I didn't realize at the time was that we were on a mission together to evolve spiritually as well.

The Fall

Lauren was in third grade now and was having Braille lessons in our home before school started. Since she was up so early, she'd typically nap as soon as she got home. I worked from home some afternoons so I could be there with her. One day she woke from a three-and-a-half-hour nap and found me in my office, down the hall from her room. She was cold so I told her to put on a robe. A few minutes later I heard a thud and then screaming. She had lost her bearings and had fallen down the stairs. She wasn't seriously hurt, but we were both terrified and I couldn't help but cry with her because it was so scary.

The next day I asked the Braille instructor if I should put up a gate. "No. Lauren needs to determine where she is," he told me.

Over the next several months, I noticed that Lauren's vision began to decrease. She'd head out to the swing set with her arms out in front of her as if she didn't want to walk into anything – a path she easily walked before. At this point, we decided she should have a cane and included that as part of her O&M therapy.

The thought of my daughter losing her vision was devastating. I was crying a lot. One night, Lauren heard me crying in my bedroom. She came in and put her arms around me, patting me on the head as I had done so many times to her. She told me gently that everything was going to be okay.

"It's not like I'm dying or anything," she said.

"You promise?"

"Yes, I plan to live a long time, mommy!" she reassured me.

I laughed and gave her a hug. She never wanted me to worry about her, but my mother's intuition told me things were not right. I had a talk with Chris the next day on the way to school. I explained to him that his sister was going to need a cane now and people may talk about her and think she is blind. I told him how sad I had been, and I expected him to feel the same way, but he surprised me.

"Life is like a road," he said, "We are all going to hit bumps. There are mountains and valleys on this road and Lauren is just climbing up a hill right now. Whatever happens, we will get through it together."

"Where'd you get so smart?" I asked and he just smiled.

I couldn't help but feel I must have done something right to have raised these two beautiful, caring and compassionate kids, both so strong and full of wisdom. I also briefly wondered what Chris' karma was; how his soul journey might fit in. For such a young boy, he certainly had a wisdom beyond his years. Could it be part of Christopher's karmic connection that he was in this family to share his wisdom and love?

CHAPTER

Ten

Unusual Times

Around age nine, Lauren started to exhibit unusual behaviors like clapping her hands and stomping her feet. Her Braille teacher said this could be something called "blindisms," which were a normal outcome of dealing with low vision. Her doctors advised us to monitor her. Over the course of a few months, the behaviors expanded to other repetitive gestures like continuously touching her thumb to her other fingers. The doctors thought she might be experiencing anxiety. In addition, the right side of her face looked like it had low-tone and she was drooling occasionally.

Lauren began sessions with a social worker for both individual and group therapy to deal with her anxiety. My husband was now away one to two weeks per month with his teaching part-time as a motivational trainer for WM, so watching for health concerns was on me. I would discuss what I saw with him. I requested that the school perform a complete psychological exam and speech tests so we could see if there was anything more concerning going on.

From the results we found she would require more speech therapy in addition to her other therapies.

The doctors agreed Lauren had lost her remaining functional vision. She was excessively tired and napping as soon as she came home from school for one to two hours. She even fell asleep in school. Things kept getting worse and I was feeling a little discouraged after all the time and effort put into conventional and alternative methods we used. I had a hard time accepting it wasn't working – at least not the way I expected. I was back to feeling like I was buying into the Emperor's New Clothes.

The Break In

It was the summer and my husband just left for one of his many two-week trips. A week had gone by, and Chris had a baseball game. I took Lauren with me to watch him play. Lauren always loved to go to these events to talk with people and visit the concession stand. A couple of hours later, I came home to find out the house had been broken into. I immediately called the police and my husband to let him know what was going on. He got on the next flight home, but wouldn't be arriving until the next day since he was on the West Coast.

I felt vulnerable and scared. I called my youngest brother, David, and he said he would come over to spend the night so we wouldn't have to be alone. He was an hour drive away, so I also called Maritza and George and they came over right away. George fixed the front door which was the entry of the break-in. He and Maritza stayed until my brother arrived. My husband arrived the next day. Once things were settled with the police and insurance, he told me he was going to leave in the morning.

"Everything is taken care of so I'm going to fly back out to teach the next class. Everything I am doing is for our family," he reminded me.

He never asked how I felt about him leaving so quickly. I felt abandoned by him. He just turned around and left! It seemed so out of the ordinary and unexpected. I felt like WM was more important than me and the needs of our family. Even when he was home, he spent lots of time on his computer, distracted and removed. I felt our relationship seemed to be the last thing he focused on. When I tried to talk to him, he said he wanted to have a better relationship but really needed to focus on being number one at WM so they would want him for their biggest and best events. He told me again and again that in the end it would be good for us.

He admitted it was hard to flip the switch when he came home. Away he was the guy on stage that everyone wanted to talk to and be with.

"At home, I'm the guy who takes out the garbage and discusses all the things that went wrong while I was away," he said.

He agreed we should have date nights and promised to be more attentive when he was home. The break-in seemed to be representative of our relationship. I not only felt robbed of my possessions, but also of a husband. It was interesting that most of the things that were taken belonged to me. My sense of security was just one of those things.

Battles on the Spiritual Front

Maritza and I spent a lot of time together over that summer. She came over almost every day to do healings and energy clearing for Lauren, which was so comforting. We both felt they were making a difference, but I wondered why Lauren was still having so many issues to confront. Everything felt like a battle, even on the spiritual front.

One night as we sat by the fire in my backyard, Maritza said, "Your father wants you to know he is connecting with healers on the other side to assist the child. His energy is persistent and determined. He is proud of the way you have been able to rise up through all the adversity you have been faced with. This is why he gave you the name 'Elizabeth,' to give you the strength and power of a queen who acts with dignity, grace and wisdom that serves her people and her family well."

Not many people know my legal name is Elizabeth since I have always been called Lisa. It was surprising and validating to have my dad come through to remind me of who I am and what my given birth name represents. I would continue to pull on that strength my dad talked about because things continued to decline for Lauren.

Third Time Around

One afternoon, she walked into a door that was normally closed and got a huge bump on her forehead. She didn't see it and we had to constantly watch her now. She also had new symptoms including uncontrollable episodes of giggling which scared the heck out of me. One night she just started pacing back and forth giggling while repeating: "Guess what Mommy, I love you. Guess what Mommy, I love you," over and over again.

My husband just held her in his arms to try and soothe her. I was a wreck and panicked over what could be causing it. I felt like my daughter was slowly slipping away from us and there was nothing we could do about it.

We took Lauren to the emergency room, and she had an EEG to check for seizures. They gave her a sedative to calm her down and did another emergency MRI. A biopsy of the tumor confirmed it was still a low-grade malignancy, but her doctors felt it was time to treat her once again with more chemo and seizure medication. It was early January of 2008 and my baby would be starting her third round of chemo with a new protocol and two new drugs. With all the symptoms Lauren was experiencing, we decided we would home school her for the remainder of fourth grade. I was allowed to work from home, but I would need help. With my husband still traveling quite a bit, I relied on Maritza, my niece, Jessica, and finally hired a "mother's helper" to watch over Lauren and help me take care of her.

Locks of Love

I had let Lauren's hair grow long since it thinned from the previous rounds of chemo. With another round of chemo coming, I talked to Lauren about how she might like a shorter haircut. Our hairdresser told Lauren about a program called Locks of Love. As soon as Lauren heard that her hair could be used to help someone else who had cancer and could give them a beautiful wig, she said, "Of course, Mommy," and was all in. She looked adorable with short hair; this would become her signature haircut. It was bob cut that was angled to be shorter in the back and longer in the front. Lauren loved the new haircut but especially loved telling everyone how she donated her hair for such a good cause.

With her new, short haircut, she was ready to face another round of chemo. At the first MRI after Lauren had begun treatment, the tumor showed a 25% reduction. She had just turned ten and it was the best birthday gift ever. The month after that her vision improved and she was able to see large letters on the CCTV (closed-circuit television) she was now using for her schoolwork. The next MRI showed further reduction of the tumor. These were the good kind of "unusuals" I welcomed any day of the week! I felt like things were finally heading in the right direction.

Just when we thought we were on an upswing, Lauren started with the giggling episodes again, and she was also drooling slightly out one side of her mouth. A scan revealed that she had developed hydrocephalus and would require a shunt surgery. That meant she had to stop chemo so they could put in this device that would allow the cerebral fluid to flow properly.

Back on the rollercoaster.

On Again Off Again

After the surgery, my husband hit the road for another workshop. People used to ask me how I felt about him traveling and leaving during such critical times and I always defended him. They didn't understand how he could leave me with all the responsibilities. "It seems unusual," they would say. At the time, I accepted it because I believed his intentions were true of doing what was best for our family in the long run. I guess I always looked at what my husband did through rose-colored glasses and assumed the best of him.

Lauren was off chemo for seven weeks before she could restart. Then she had three weeks of chemo before more symptoms appeared and she needed a second shunt. That meant chemo had to stop once more so she could prep for another surgery and recovery afterward. This time it was eight weeks before she could restart.

It was now December of 2008 and the next MRI showed the tumor had grown twenty-five to thirty percent and Lauren's team of doctors felt the chemo was not working. They wanted to stop treatment. I protested because she had such great results early on.

"It grew because she's been off chemo for 13 weeks with two shunt surgeries!" I said. Surely, they could see that and would agree this protocol was working for her, but they did not and the treatment stopped.

Hawaii Here We Come

Fortunately, during the next several months Lauren's MRIs were all stable. We decided it was time to take an amazing family vacation to regroup after all the surgeries and chemo. We asked Chris and Lauren, "If you could go anywhere in the world where would that be?" Lauren suggested Hawaii and Chris agreed it was a great idea. So, for April spring break we planned a ten-day trip to the Hawaiian Islands. Chris was twelve and half and Lauren just turned eleven. It would be a great family trip that they would both remember!

We asked Maritza if she would like to come with us on the trip. It would serve as a thank you for all the help she provided over the years. She was not only a great friend but also a healer to Lauren. At first, she didn't want to impose but I told her she would be an added help with Lauren when she wanted to rest or if she was unable to make an excursion that we wanted to do with Chris. She gladly accepted and it was a wonderful trip. We went to the Big Island and Maui and there was so much for all of us to do and see.

One day when we took Chris on a helicopter excursion to see a volcano, Lauren and Maritza stayed behind and went to the pool. It was a big resort and Maritza couldn't figure out how to get back to the room.

"I'm so sorry, Lauren, but I'm lost," she said. "Your parents are going to be so mad at me."

"It's okay," Lauren said. "Let's just stop for a minute and take a breath and I know we will find it. And don't worry, this will be our secret."

Lauren was so happy to have little secrets like that. She never did tell me. I only found out when I asked Maritza to share a story she remembers from that trip.

Maritza and I will never forget the night we all went to a luau. Of course, Lauren wanted to speak to as many people as she could. Even though she needed a cane to get around and could only see a few feet in front of her, it didn't stop her from talking to just about everyone. A beautiful Hawaiian woman approached us and asked if it was okay if she spoke with Lauren.

She held Lauren's hand and gazed at her with these amazing eyes that sparkled as she spoke softly to her. After she walked away, Maritza told me she felt her strong energy and knew she was a healer. We wondered if she was doing energy work on Lauren. I immediately felt compelled to speak with her about it, but it was as if she had disappeared. We looked all around for her, but she was nowhere to be found. It was so odd.

We felt the amazing healing energy that night and at other places across the island. It was especially high near the grounds of King Kamehameha and at the pools of Ohe'o, better known as The Seven Healing Pools you can find on the road to Hana. We stopped at so many beautiful waterfalls along the way and of course placed some of the sacred water from each of the seven pools on Lauren's face and body. Lauren had developed a heightened sense of hearing and she could hear the waterfalls before we could. She would say: "Listen, do you hear that?" It was such a peaceful sound and Maritza reminded us to never underestimate the healing power of water.

The Deeper Mind

That summer I decided to get my certification in hypnotherapy from Pathways. Hypnosis teaches you about how the deeper mind works and included a session on how to do past life regressions. By taking this certification, I learned even more about the mind, body and spirit connection. The main reason why I did this was to further assist my girl. Taking hypnotherapy also validated my earlier findings with Maritza regarding past lives.

Dr. Bezmen explained how the subconscious mind is like a vast computer with memory banks that hold every event, every thought, every emotion and every place the subject has experienced in this lifetime and prior. In order for healing to occur, it is necessary to tap into the knowledge stored in the subconscious mind and to bring this information into conscious awareness. By doing this, we can release or diffuse the energy and emotional blockages that keep us stuck and cause us to repeat patterns. To heal the present, it is important to first resolve unfinished business from the past. The events from the past continue to create an emotional charge upon us until they are released or cleared.

I couldn't do past life regression with Lauren because she was too young, but I could use guided visualization to help create safe and beautiful places for her to go to while she was having intense treatments such as chemo, MRIs and surgeries. What first felt somewhat bizarre became techniques I would count on to calm and comfort my child.

As my husband continued to increase his traveling and teaching for WM, he was thinking about doing it full time. He felt he had found his calling and loved being on stage. It would mean he'd be away even more. He hired an associate doctor to cover his practice full-time so he could focus on his professional speaker/trainer career. More and more opportunities were coming his way and with Lauren now stable, it was a good time for him to explore those options.

Brownie Sundae Saga

One of Lauren's favorite places to go was Friendly's restaurant. She especially loved to order the mac and cheese and, of course, ice cream. Our good friend, Trish, who has been friends with my husband since they were children, liked to take her there. One time, my husband showed up when they were ordering dessert. They all ordered brownie sundaes. He ordered his with "the works" and when he was finished, he got up and left without paying.

"How dare he do that?" Trish joked.

"Seriously!" Lauren said as she rolled her eyes up to the ceiling.

"Well, now he owes you a brownie sundae," Lauren added.

It was always amazing how this little one who was losing her vision used her eyes so expressively. From then on, the brownie sundae saga was a standing joke with Lauren always reminding her father that he owed Trish a brownie sundae.

"I don't remember it happening like that. Trish owes *me* a brownie sundae!" He would say.

Lauren's mouth would drop open and the look on her face was always priceless. Lauren had a great sense of humor and liked to tease, just like her dad did. In fact, playfully teasing and tormenting was his signature way of interacting with her.

It also became Lauren's way of interacting with others – including Trish's husband Dan, although more affectionately.

"Your nickname is King Commander Master Handsome Cool Dude!" she proclaimed during one of their phone conversations. As she grew older and grew closer with Trish, she would tell Dan he was still the King, but Trish was the Queen and he had to massage her and "run, not walk" whenever she needed something. This was Lauren's quirky sense of humor.

The Apron and the Bell

I think around this time Lauren came up with another brilliant idea, which I call "The Apron and The Bell." Lauren would tell men that they needed to give their wives or girlfriend a bell, and they should wear an apron. Anytime their lady needed something, she could ring the bell and he should run (not walk) to see what they needed. This became a priceless bit of wisdom Lauren would share and it would have us all rolling. The way Lauren said things and the funny faces she made were hilarious.

Do the Dance

All Lauren wanted to do was laugh and play like every other child. Even though she had limited vision, she loved watching T.V. too, especially shows like American Idol and America's Funniest Home Videos where she could easily understand what was happening from listening. One of her favorite episodes on Funniest Home Videos was when a wife locked her husband outside in the rain and wouldn't let him back in until he did a dance. She thought that was an excellent idea and whenever she had the opportunity, she would lock someone out of the car, house or wherever and then she'd say: "Do the dance." I have to admit she'd mostly torture her dad this way. The best part was seeing how much she enjoyed it.

She also liked to watch sitcoms and movies that made her laugh and stole lines from them. When she watched Full House, she started saying: "How rude!" and "You got it, dude!" From the movie Freaky Friday, she would say: "UH, you're ruining my life" whenever she was annoyed with me. Lauren became a keen listener, and it was funny that she grabbed on to lines from both T.V. shows and commercials. I joined in and would tell her each morning: "It's Time to Make the Donuts" when she didn't want to get out of bed.

I also got really good at finding tactile or sound-based games we could play. I found Braille Go Fish cards online and we made a tabletop box she could hold her cards under (so no one else could see them). Lauren loved arts and crafts, so I worked with her to cover the box with beautiful pink material and decorated it with rhinestones with her initials on it. We played Go Fish almost every night after dinner. Her brother used to say she cheated all the time. She did like to win, and I actually think the little stinker kept extra cards underneath the table on her lap. Her dad would usually play a game or two with her before he dived into his computer for the rest of the night preparing or planning for his next training event.

It was so great to have these "normal" family times amongst all the "unusual" times we had come to accept as our normal. Her brother always saw Lauren as his sister – not a sick child or girl losing her vision, just his sister, and she always saw him as her big brother whom she adored. Just like any brother and sister they did their share of teasing each other but there was a very strong bond between them. She always wanted to know where her brother was and enjoyed hanging out with him and his friends when they came over until they were ready to go in the basement and play video games or some other activity.

A Teacher's Gift

Lauren would be starting sixth grade in the fall and her teacher, Mrs. H, unexpectedly called asking to visit. We were delighted by her effort to get to know Lauren and understand her needs before the school year began. During her visit, she brought Lauren a gift. It was a beautiful textured box with perfume sprayed on the inside. She told Lauren to smell inside and whenever she smells that at school, Lauren would know she was nearby. Not only was this exceptional but she also brought her kids with her who were in Lauren's grade to allow her to meet some classmates in advance.

While Lauren was excited and well prepared to start school, she was very tired in the afternoons. It was clear she could only manage attending half days so I worked with Mrs. H to set up her schedule so she got all her academics covered in the morning. Then she could come home and nap before having an afternoon full of therapies.

I was able to leave work early and work from home in the afternoons which allowed me to talk with her therapists and keep a close eye on how Lauren was doing. I also wanted to reassure Lauren that mommy was there for her. Lauren was usually never far from me no matter what. I used to joke how she would even follow me into the bathroom, and I would have to say, "Excuse me, but can I have a minute?" I became an expert at balancing her needs, work and the rest of our home life. It was a collaborative effort and could not have been accomplished without the help of Lauren's teachers and faculty at the Miller Place school district who were all incredible!

Reflections of ME

Naturally, Lauren's favorite class at school was art. That year she worked on a special project called "Reflections of Me," a collage of all her favorite things. She included her hand prints; some of her favorite foamies; her special star, butterfly and heart beads; and wrappers from her favorite Werther candies. It was so beautiful, colorful and sparkled just like she did.

Reflecting back on these extraordinarily unusual times, I can also see all the extraordinary and exceptional people who touched her life – and in turn our lives. I recognize these people were all reflections of Lauren and her uplifting attitude and spirit. She drew most people in like a magnet and they became enriched by this extraordinary little girl who rose up beyond each and every challenge she faced in her life.

It was touching that her "Reflections of ME" art project was selected to appear in the Stony Brook Museum of Art that Christmas. Little did we know where we would be at that time.

CHAPTER

Eleven

Six Weeks Turn To Six Months

Not long after school started, I noticed Lauren was having some balance issues so I was keeping a close eye on her. One afternoon, we were standing in the kitchen and Lauren was right next to me when she just collapsed. At first, I thought she was kidding around but a second later I realized this was serious. My husband was away. When I called him, he told me to stay calm. "The doctor said not to worry about anything unless there is a pattern," he said.

I called the doctor anyway, but he agreed with my husband. "Let's just monitor her for now," he said.

When my husband returned home, she collapsed a second time and luckily, I was able to break her fall. I was pretty upset and wanted to take her for an emergency MRI.

"It isn't a predictable pattern. No need to rush to the hospital," my husband said.

Then, almost as he was speaking, she collapsed again in front of both us.

"Now can we take her to the ER?" I asked.

We immediately called the doctors and decided to take her to New York University Hospital (NYUH) in Manhattan where they had an entire NF1 speciality team.

Lauren's CT (cat scan) results indicated the shunt was malfunctioning and they needed to perform a shunt revision. The surgery would fix the device that drained fluid from her brain to her stomach. After a few days in the hospital, things looked a little better.

They sent us home, but Lauren continued to have balance issues. We went back and forth to the city almost every week for several weeks to have MRIs and meetings with NF specialists. It was a two-hour ride each way and were very draining days. Our new oncologist conferred with a pediatric neurosurgeon and suggested it might be time for a tumor resection. The tumor had progressively grown over the last eight years and was sizable.

Symptoms First

Now I understood why Lauren's speech was slurred and why she was weak on the entire right side of her body. She was displaying limited use of her hand and arm and was starting to walk with a little bit of a limp for some time now. They called this right-sided hemiparesis due to brain injury from the tumor on the left side of her brain.

124

Research showed that NF1 tumors typically stopped growing at age six, but Lauren was now eleven and it was obviously steadily progressing. I always saw physical signs something was wrong before the MRI confirmed the tumor was on the move or changing shape. It was clear this was causing her serious issues and taking away from her quality of life.

It would be a risky surgery – any type of brain surgery is – and while the doctors could not guarantee results, they felt this was the best option for Lauren. The goal would be to remove as much of the tumor as possible without endangering her. It would be (approximately) a five-hour surgery and about six weeks of recovery in the rehab center, which was adjacent to the hospital.

I had a friend at work who had a son with a brain tumor. He saw the same pediatric oncologist and neurologist as Lauren and had gone through many procedures. It was reassuring to speak with her and listen to her calm approach.

"How do you get through it?" I asked her.

"Lisa, we just take everything one day and one surgery at a time," she said. That was the approach I would adopt as well.

One of the weirdest things to witness was the prep for Lauren's surgery. They placed green plastic markers all over her head so the neurosurgeon could see exactly where the tumor was during surgery in case it shifted since the last MRI. We were shown how he would operate with a real-time imaging machine and the markers would be precise indicators of where it was. It was surreal to see and I had a new appreciation of what technology can do.

I kept looking at my beautiful baby girl wondering if this would be the last time she would remember me. They said they couldn't guarantee the outcome and I was frightened that this might be the last time I would ever see my Lauren. It was another one of those life-altering, pivotal moments and I had no idea or control over what was about to happen. I had to keep a brave face on for my girl and hold back my tears though they wanted to burst out of me.

Lauren was incredibly brave. Even with the markers all over her head, to her this was just another surgery and was comforted by having her family all around her. I couldn't stop kissing her and hugging her while we waited for them to prep her. I was always the one to go into the operating room with her and stay until she was sleeping comfortably from the anesthesia. This time I lingered longer than usual. The OR staff told me it was finally time to leave. Please take care of my beautiful baby girl I said to them as I gave Lauren one more kiss on her forehead and told her I love her.

Five Hours Later

It was the longest day of my life. My mom and my husband's parents were with us in the waiting room as four, then five hours passed with no sign of the surgeon. I was getting more and more worried by the minute and there was nothing I could do. My superhero suit was of no use to me – I had to take the fear that engulfed me, and just let it be. There was nothing to do but wait and I struggled. I had to remind myself to breathe as I waited.

"They said four to five hours," I said. "Where are they? What's happening?"

Every minute was another minute of agony. I paced from the coffee machine to the couch where everyone was sitting.

The surgeon finally came out five and half hours later and sat us in a private room to tell us the surgery was a success. He felt he was able to remove thirty to fifty percent of the tumor.

"Thank you, God!" I said.

I was so relieved to hear this news and anxious to see my Lauren. She slept the rest of the day and night. I prayed in the chair next to her to bed the entire time. I can't tell you how happy I was when she opened her eyes the next morning and said her first word, "Mommy."

"Oh my God, you're OK!"

As the day progressed, she ate Jell-O and drank water and we were elated that she had no problems with her memory or speech.

My husband and I both stayed by her side day and night. Only one of us could sleep in the chair next to her bed, so the other slept on a couch in the parent room down the hall. Neither one of us got much sleep, but at least there was a place to shower and change our clothes. After a week, a social worker helped arranged for us to get into the Ronald McDonald House across town and I was the first one to go over there to get a good night's rest.

When I came back the next morning, my husband told me about a moment in the early morning when he wanted to leave Lauren's room to shave but a nurse stopped him at the door and asked him to wait. He wondered why. As he watched, a stretcher with a body covered by a sheet rolled by. Judging by the patient's size, he guessed it was a child about the same age as Lauren.

127

"In that moment I was so grateful for everything, including the surgeries Lauren had gone through the past week, the ventilator tube she'd had in her mouth, the five IV lines, the catheter, the sleepless nights, the crappy hospital food – and most of all, Lauren," he said.

An event like that puts everything into proper perspective. I gave him a hug and told him how grateful I was for everything too.

L A U R E N   R O C K S

To keep busy, there were child life therapists that did arts and crafts, played games and music with all the children on the floor. My husband spent his time making big block letters with Lauren that he taped up to the window in her room so you could easily see from outside the hospital that said: L A U R E N   R O C K S!

A few weeks later, Lauren moved to RUSK, the rehab wing at NYUH to regain her strength and start the necessary therapies. Over the next several weeks she suffered shunt complications, possibly from surgical debris, and she would require more surgeries to clear blockages. It happened so many times I almost lost count. Normally, you give your room up in rehab if you move back to the hospital, but Lauren went back and forth so many times they saved the bed in her room. I did my best to make the small space they gave her cozy. I decorated her wall with a blue sky and clouds and posted all the cards people were sending and we called it the "Carden" instead of a garden. We would read them to her as they arrived and posted them on her wall.

The room had four other young girls each recovering from something different. Each girl had her own space divided by nothing more than a thin curtain. Trying to rest in the sleeper chair next to

Lauren's bed was nearly impossible as you could hear the beeping and alerts all night long for all five girls. One child had to get a shot every morning, and she'd scream in terror at the top of her lungs. That was our wake-up call each morning.

There was so much going on with Lauren it was hard to keep everyone informed. I repeated the same information over and over. My sister, Annalise, helped me update Lauren's website, LaurensVision.com, to add a blog page so I could keep family and friends informed about her hospital stay. I included pictures along with reports about how she was doing.

Dr. McDreamy

With all the surgeries Lauren was having, we got to know some of the doctors and nurses pretty well. There were two young neurosurgeon residents that Lauren took a liking to. One was tall and handsome and always spoke in a soft gentle voice. She called him Dr. McDreamy and said it in a dreamy way. The other doctor was more to the point but always very nice and he would ask her, "What's my name?" to which Lauren replied, "You're just Todd," and then she would laugh. It was hilarious because all the nurses swooned over Dr. McDreamy and it was uncanny how Lauren seemed to sense he was a handsome man. From then on, the nurses all called the other doctor "Just Todd" which he had Lauren to thank for.

She was such a trooper in the hospital. No matter how many times they came in to take blood, put in an IV or poke her for one thing or the other, she was always brave. Whenever anyone asked her how she was doing, she always answered "Grreeeaaatttt!" She said this even when I knew she wasn't feeling so great, but that was my girl. Everyone commented how amazing it was that Lauren remained so happy and positive despite all she was going through.

Happy, Positive and Healthy

One morning when the docs, including Dr. McDreamy, came in to do their rounds, they asked Lauren the same question they asked her every day, "So, Miss Lauren how are you feeling today?"

"I'm HPH!" she said.

I looked at her and asked, "What does HPH stand for?"

"It means Happy, Positive and Healthy!" she said.

"You certainly are!" I said. From her lips to God's ears, I prayed.

Lauren would continue to use HPH from that day forward to describe how she felt and was another way she displayed her incredible positive disposition.

Double Trouble

It was four weeks in at the hospital and we thought Lauren was turning a corner with the shunts when we were hit with more bad news. An MRI showed that the tumor had doubled in size. The team wanted to do a second tumor resection.

"How is that even possible?" I asked her doctor.

"Sometimes tumors can retaliate in response to a resection, or it could be that it was so tightly compressed that once there was more space in the brain, the tumor had room to unravel." Another long brain surgery was scheduled for New Year's Eve.

Once more I found myself pacing outside the OR waiting room. Everyone we knew had prayer chains going for Lauren, extending all around the world. The doc came out some five hours later to tell us the surgery was a success. They would have to do a biopsy on the tumor to determine why it grew so rapidly, and then they would discuss next steps with us.

The biopsy revealed the tumor was still a junior polycystic astrocytoma (JPA), which meant it was not malignant. These classifications had to do with how rapidly the tumor cells divide. Regardless, they wanted to do twenty-eight days of radiation to ensure it would not grow radically again. Lauren woke up the next morning again and recovered even quicker than she did the first time. It felt like a miracle, and I continued to thank God for the blessings as they came.

Meals on Wheels

Back at home, word got out that we were going to be in the hospital longer than expected. A wonderful woman named Marian, who was a girl scout leader in our town, offered to arrange meals for us for as long as we needed. She reached out to our neighbors and organized this act of love and had folks sign up to prepare and deliver meals to our doorstep. We gratefully accepted, knowing we'd be running back and forth from NYUH and not have much time to shop and prepare meals. We had no idea just how long we would be utilizing this act of neighborly love adding it to the things we would be grateful for.

Both of our families were helping to take care of Chris at home and bringing him to the hospital to see Lauren. My husband and I stayed by Lauren's side until we were sure things were under control. I took family medical leave for three months, never imagining her stay would go beyond that.

Back and Forth We Go

I wish I could tell you things went fine after the second resection – but she kept having shunt complications that delayed radiation. Lauren went back and forth from the ICU (intensive care unit) to rehab for the better part of six months. She was so tired she could barely participate in all the therapies required for her rehabilitation. She continued to be such a trooper and gave it everything she had. But more than anything she just wanted to come home.

I was still working with holistic practitioners and had met someone new right before Lauren's hospitalization. Her name was Lynne and she was an energy healer. Her boyfriend, Derek, was a Shaman. I took Lauren to see them a couple of months before the tumor resection and they both did healing work on her.

Lynne came to the hospital once a week the entire six months Lauren was there. She worked with crystal bowls which harmonize with the body's chakras. She would bring the bowls to the hospital and play them for Lauren to assist in her healing. It was soothing to hear them played and Lauren enjoyed Lynne's visits as much as the sound of the crystal bowls.

Lauren was finally ready to start radiation and I used guided visualizations from my hypnotherapy training to help put Lauren (and me) in a calm state. She had to wear a mesh mask over her face, which was secured to the table beneath her so she couldn't move while she received radiation. This would be enough to give any adult or child anxiety and I feared Lauren might go into a panic while this was going on. I wasn't allowed to be in the room but could stand right outside and speak to her through a microphone.

I had a ritual we did as they prepared everything for radiation. I explained and described everything that was going on around her and put on her favorite music. When everything was set up, I would start a gentle guided meditation from inside the room holding her hand. Once I was sure she was calm and in a relaxed state I moved outside the room and continued the meditation on a microphone in the technician area and continued throughout the radiation treatment.

I just wanted to keep her calm and assured that I was right there with her. It was horrifying to see my baby on a table unable to move with this mask covering her face. The meditation did its trick and she stayed calm for each and every treatment.

It was a long twenty-eight days. On the last day of treatment, the two young women who were her radiation technicians got Lauren a stuffed build-a-bear in hospital clothes to cheer her on with her recovery. Between all the surgeries Lauren had gone through plus the radiation, she was very weak. She had lost a lot of weight and was barely 100 pounds.

Forgotten Birthday

Toward the end of her stay Lauren was sometimes able to come home on the weekends if her blood work was okay. We all looked forward to that. Medical bills were piling up and my family medical leave was also up. I worked out an arrangement that I could work four long days a week and take Friday off so I could get back to the hospital. My husband stayed with Lauren Monday through Thursday and I would get there late Thursday night and stay until Sunday night. This way one parent could be with Lauren and one with Chris. We had to keep up with things like his dentist appointments, schoolwork, school trips, and sports.

Occasionally my husband and I got to go out for a bite to eat when we changed shifts at the hospital, as long as another family member or friend was visiting and could stay with her. In the midst of this crazy and stressful time, apparently we all forgot his birthday. He never said anything until long after, and kind of made a joke about it.

"Aw, Babe, I'm so sorry, why didn't you say anything sooner?"

I couldn't believe I actually would have forgotten his birthday, but I also couldn't remember if we had done anything to celebrate or at least had said Happy Birthday. Life was spinning out of control then. Regardless, he would never let me or anyone else ever forget that we forgot his birthday.

Fundraiser

Lauren would be spending her twelfth birthday in the hospital with no estimation of when she might be able to leave. Our friend, Trish, decided to do something special for the whole family and put together a fundraiser to help out with all the medical costs and other expenses we were incurring. She had done large fundraisers for her church and was well experienced. My youngest sister, Cathy, was bartending at a popular pub in Wantagh, and they offered us the use of their place for free. My older sister, Marion, led the effort to make the baskets and solicit for prizes. The rest of my family and other friends helped out on the day of the event.

There was an amazing turnout and though Lauren was supposed to be there, the week before the event she experienced another complication and then more surgery. Thanks to technology, she made an appearance via Skype and the crowd cheered! People were so generous and kind to us at the event and for that, we are forever grateful.

The hospital is also filled with amazing people. Doctors, nurses, therapists, social workers and other health care workers – all really caring people. Then there are the volunteers. People who show up with presents for children in the ICU at Christmas time, clowns and other entertainers who just want to help your child smile – all completely PRICELESS. The clown at NYUH named "Looney Lenny" would always tease Lauren and pretend to never get her name right. He would call her "Snorin" or "Pouren" and then finally called her Snorin Lauren, which she hated. She would tease him right back and all the kids would think this was hilarious.

Do Not What?

One day when it was my turn to be with Lauren, she exhibited concerning symptoms. I discussed them with the nurse on duty. She and I were friendly and she knew to trust my instincts, so she alerted the doctor on call.

I suspected Lauren was having another shunt malfunction, but it was late and the resident said we would just monitor her through the night and do surgery in the morning if necessary. We were moved to the ICU and got settled. I was sleeping next to Lauren when all of a sudden, alarms started going off. Before I knew it, there were half a dozen nurses and doctors rushing in. I had no idea what was happening.

One of the nurses ushered me outside Lauren's room while more doctors rushed in.

"Have you signed a DNR?"

"Wait, what? You want to know if I signed a Do Not Resuscitate?" I was confused. "If you're telling me that she is in critical condition, you better get her oncologist and neurosurgeon here right now!"

Everything was happening so fast but felt like I was watching in slow motion. I saw them put paddles on her chest and her little body jumped and then I knew exactly what was happening. She must have flat-lined. They waited too long and now her life was at risk. I couldn't believe what was happening. I stood outside her room, motionless. Finally, they stabilized her and prepped her for immediate surgery.

I rushed back to her side and held her hand until they took her for yet another shunt revision. The count was reaching two dozen surgeries since she came to the hospital. After they took her to the operating room, I found my way to a chapel/meditation room in the hospital. I sat there and cried and then prayed to God that he would give us both the strength and grace to make it through all of this.

By now, God and I were well acquainted, and I invited God into my life often. I was cultivating our relationship, trying to figure out our communication. I believed in miracles and prayed for them. The miracle I wanted was for Lauren to be well – no more tumor, full strength in her body and her vision restored. *"Ask and it is given,"* the Bible says. I was on my knees in that chapel as I asked and prayed for that and kept a hopeful heart.

I left the chapel with swollen eyes and started to make my way back to Lauren's hospital room. I walked down the hallway numb with a glazed look on my face as I entertained the thought of, "How could this all be happening to us?" And more importantly, "Why?"

CHAPTER

Twelve

Faith, Family & Friends

I don't how any of us would have gotten through these trying times, especially the hospital days, without our faith, family and friends. All played a huge role in keeping me grounded and, quite frankly, from losing my mind. My faith kept me especially centered when everything was falling apart around me. It could only have been God's grace that we got through it all.

Invite God In

I listened to Joel Osteen often and found much comfort in his words. I remember when he spoke about inviting God into your difficulties. He said sometimes the miracle is not in getting *out*, it's what God is going to do for you while *in* the situation. He suggested praying for God to come in wherever you are to help you shine bright and be your best.

"Always shine your light," he would say.

So I prayed for God's light to be present while Lauren was receiving her chemo or medication to guide it to be absorbed by her body to make her well. I also prayed for God to be present in the operating room and guide the hands of the surgeon. I especially prayed for God to give me the strength and grace to cope with all that was happening to my baby girl. I can tell you that I did receive strength that I could not explain and grace to outlast what brought me to my knees. There was great power in prayer for me. It changed me and allowed me to deepen my faith. A faith that would guide me and serve me for a long time to come. A faith I would share with Lauren, which helped us both not just go through, but grow through, the rough times.

Maritza was a huge comfort to me and would recite her favorite Bible passages. She reminded me that God would be with us when we go through the river or a fire – not necessarily keep us from it. When things got really rough, she told me she always went to her favorite scripture, Psalm 23, and it became my favorite too.

Peaks And Valleys

I have to say that it was during the times in the valley that I deepened my faith. It was a great comfort to know that I was not alone. Though I could not see a way, surely God had a way out of the valley and would always lead me to green pastures and still waters.

"Without a great test, you can't have great testimony," Joel Osteen would say. I kept my faith and hope that all was at work for our highest good. I imagined the amazing testimony we would have and could see my husband telling it from the stage when this was all behind us.

I felt it was God that held me up when I could not stand and gave me the strength I needed to get through. I believe that God's love is with me and all around me and shows up in the *people* that show up in our life. I believe the creator of the universe provides the power to overcome what *should* stop you. There's no other way to explain it.

I was also told over and over again that things don't happen on our timetable but in God's time. So, I would wait and pray and believe that all would be well. Even so, I still had the tendency to fight for what I wanted, to argue, even with Spirit when things didn't go the way I wanted. I used to joke with Maritza that even with the spirits there's always a back door, another avenue to try.

Hope

Joyce Meyer is a practical bible teacher on television that I related to very much. She inspired me and helped me get through some of my most difficult days.

"Hope is the happy anticipation of good. Hope releases JOY. Hope is a positive attitude. The hopeful person refuses to be negative in any way, although they recognize and deal with the storms of life, they remain hopeful in thought, attitude and in their conversation," she said during one of her broadcasts.

I called her Mama Joyce and liked when she said we can't live by how we feel and what we see. If you have a thought that makes you feel bad, just change your thought and your feelings will catch back up with you, she would preach. When you expect something bad to happen, it usually does and likewise, if you expect something good to happen, it eventually comes. It reconfirmed what I already knew and helped me wake up with a positive attitude that every day is an opportunity for something new and possibly better to happen.

"What are you expecting God to do in your life?" Joyce would ask. "You don't hope for what you can see or already have, you hope for what you can't see and what you don't have."

My hopes and expectations were set on the full recovery for Lauren. Since I knew many healers and intuitives, there were times I asked what message they had for me about all Lauren was going through. It usually brought comfort to me. I found myself always asking "Why?" I just needed things to make sense. Plenty of times I asked different healers and psychics the same questions, waiting to get the answers that made sense to me or maybe what I wanted to hear.

Maritza would shake her head at me. "It doesn't work that way," she would remind me. Even though I had my questions, I believed God always gave me faith, grace and strength. Faith gave me hope. Grace gave me calm and peace. Strength gave me the power to push on. Without all of which, I would have certainly fallen apart.

Loving Her Through

In addition to having to recover from all of her surgeries, Lauren was suffering from post-radiation exhaustion and was sleeping most of the day as well as the night and could not participate in the acute rehab at Rusk Center at NYU. It was a requirement that you could actively participate in at least four hours of therapy to stay in the program. Lauren did not have the strength for it.

142

After six months at the hospital, the medical director told us the best thing for Lauren was to let her get rest in the comfort of her home. She was discharged on May 6, 2010. My husband and I were not quite sure how we were going to take care of Lauren and manage all she needed. She did not have the strength to walk, talk, see or even turn herself in bed. But we were determined to do all that we could for our little angel.

Love and support from our family and friends is what got us through the following year. Everyone we knew, and some we didn't, helped us love Lauren through this rough time. People used to say, "I don't know how you do it." Honestly, I don't know either. I just did whatever needed to get done.

Making It Work

It was the same at work and I truly believe my experience working as a program manager for a global IT (information technology) company helped prepare me for what was to come. At work my job was to find out what was required, manage the process and team, set milestones, measure success and report on progress. I was used to working under extreme pressure and managing relationships with a variety of people at various levels in the organization from all over the world. I continued to work full time and had a manager during this time who was not so understanding and required me to be at the office. It was difficult to leave my little girl during the day, but I needed to work because I carried the benefits and made good money. There were times I broke down and cried at my desk or in the bathroom and was thankful I had my friend Lisa there to comfort me.

My husband still had a doctor covering at his chiropractic office and could be with Lauren most days, but he was looking forward to getting back to the world of professional speaking since he had put it on hold for six months. We had a hospital bed in our living room so we could watch Lauren every minute during the day, and I slept on the couch to be with her through the night. Slowly she began to regain her strength. She could sit up with support, but she had different issues popping up.

Maritza came over almost every day to help out and so did my niece Jessica. This provided much needed relief and allowed us to take care of other things. The biggest hurdle was to get Lauren enrolled in Medicaid. This took many months of working with a social worker from the hospital to get it set up. She couldn't get any assistance until that was done. Bills were mounting with only me working and made me anxious.

Lauren also started a new immuno-therapy, so there were ongoing doctor visits and treatments to follow up on. We had to travel back and forth from Long Island to New York University Hospital (NYUH), which was over a two hour ride each way. She needed a custom wheelchair, and we had to buy a new car to make accommodations for that and to make it easier for Lauren to get in and out. The money from the fundraiser came in handy for both these things.

As she started moving around, Lauren had fainting episodes that were so crazy. One minute she would be fine and the next minute, she would drop. The docs said it appeared to be an effect from spending so much time lying down. They called it vasovagal syncope. She would faint if she got up too quickly, but would also happen sometimes when she laughed. In addition, she had trouble drinking liquids. All her drinks had to be thickened so she wouldn't choke. It was scary stuff to take care of her on our own and this would go on for the better part of the year.

Surprise

My sister Cathy was getting married in June, the month after Lauren got out of the hospital. She and her fiancé Bryan, whom Lauren loved, were having a destination wedding in Jamaica. My sister had ordered Lauren a special dress, hoping she could be in the bridal party since she was such a special part of their lives. Lauren desperately wanted to go. After a lot of debate, we agreed Lauren was still too weak to travel so I made travel arrangements for me and Chris.

In Jamaica on the day before the wedding, I was working out early in the morning with my niece, Jessica, when I got a call. The hotel receptionist said there was a special gift for me in the lobby. I ran over to see what it was and there was my husband with Lauren in her wheelchair!

"What are you guys doing here?" I asked while staring at my husband.

"I took Lauren to Friendly's to have dinner and she was just so sad," he said. "I decided right then and there to see if I could make it happen."

He explained that he called Lauren's doctors and got the okay to take her. He immediately booked their flights. She was so happy and so was everyone else. We got our room upgraded to be on the first floor, near the wedding reception so Lauren could rest whenever she needed to.

"You look like handsome love," she told Bryan, the groom. She beamed with happiness that she was able to be at this joyous occasion with FAMILY – which we all needed!

CHAPTER

Thirteen

My Girls

It would take five months before we got Medicaid approved and the first thing Lauren qualified for was a home nurse. Lauren was completely blind at this point and needed assistance with all her daily living activities, not to mention the concerns with fainting and choking she was still having. We went through a couple of nurses before we finally found someone who we felt was competent to handle all of Lauren's needs. Carly was a young nurse in her twenties who was confident, beautiful and kind. She had long blonde hair and always wore her make-up perfectly, wearing her signature pink lipstick every day. She would grow to become one of Lauren's closest friends, confidantes and fashion coordinator.

Having a nurse during the week was so helpful and reassuring. Carly was great with Lauren, who loved having someone new to talk to. It would take several more months before we got approval to hire home health aides. But once we got that, life would greatly improve for all of us. It was challenging for me to work all day and then take care of Lauren in the evening and weekends and I was feeling the effects. It reminded me of having an infant, only with Lauren there was no telling how long it could go on.

New BFFs

Once we got the approval for aides, the agency gave the option to send people over or you could hire and manage them yourself. Since I was pretty selective about who I wanted in our home helping Lauren, I opted for the latter. I got a system down where I looked for competent college students who were going to school for nursing or a related health field, who could not only help take care of Lauren, but also be a friend to her. Someone who had compassion as well as a sense of humor and who could fit into our family. I was blessed to find one lovely girl after another.

All the girls got very close to Lauren and to me. She loved them all; there was something very special about each and every one. Carly spent the most time with Lauren and I am grateful for her and her influence on Lauren. Yes, it was Carly's job to look after her as a nurse, but it was so much more than that. She became a big sister to Lauren, and they had fun together. Carly was a bit of a fashionista and taught Lauren the importance of putting outfits together and accessorizing with pocketbooks and jewelry. It brightened her day each time Carly came through the door and said, "Hey Lau" in her sweet and caring voice.

Amanda was the first aide I hired. She was only eighteen. She had long dark hair, was sweet, kind and spoke in a very gentle soft voice. Lauren instantly liked her.

"Oh, Lauren," she would say with her sweet giggle in reply to all the funny things Lauren said. Amanda couldn't fill all the hours and so she recommended her friend Brittany to help out. Brittany brought a little different energy into the house. As soon as she came through the door, she'd shout, "Hey-Hey-Heyy!" Since these two girls were friends, whenever they crossed shifts, they would stay for a bit and chat. Lauren loved that and felt like it was a girl party. She got to talk to exhaustion and ask these girls everything about their lives.

"What color is your hair?" She would ask them all. "May I feel how long it is?"

Lauren had new best friends and was influenced by these girls. She decided she wanted to go blonde like Carly and asked me she could have her hair highlighted.

"That takes a really long time to sit still in a chair," I told her.

"I don't care, I'll do it," she said.

It's funny how this child who could not see insisted on getting blonde highlights and was willing to sit in the chair at the hairdresser for hours every few months. I think she enjoyed all the compliments she got from the girls and how everyone raved how great she looked.

Boyfriends were another big topic and she got to live vicariously through their experiences, not just with boys but also with school, work, family and other friends. These girls brought so much joy, laughter and fun back into Lauren's life and our home.

Team Lauren

There would be many aides that would come and go, but some would be very special girls who brought their unique sense of humor, friendship and love. I felt so blessed to find such wonderful help who found their way into our hearts and our home. Once again proving "it takes a village" and I found how true this was over and over again. I could not do everything myself to take care of Lauren, but with the help of these girls, or as I liked to call them "My Girls," we did it. They became part of the larger "Team Lauren" along with her teachers, doctors and therapists.

As Lauren regained her strength, it was time to bring therapists back in. She needed more PT, OT and speech therapy. I took this on to research and find the right people. I would also coordinate all the scheduling of her sessions. It was right up my alley.

We also had to make some accommodations in the house and redid the bathrooms to suit Lauren's needs. The kids' bathroom was completely redone to accommodate rolling a wheelchair into the shower and under the sink area. We installed motion faucets to make things easier for her and to allow her to have as much independence as possible. That fall, Lauren started homeschooling and we got the good news that the tumor had shrunk by seventy-five percent. Yay!

Most of Lauren's teachers and therapists were amazing. Those that weren't, I replaced. I probably had a reputation at school because of how involved and demanding I was, but Lauren needed a lot of support to get back on track and I was going to be sure she got what she needed. What I didn't know was behind the scenes there was a lot of debate on whether or not to give Lauren all the things she required. It was expensive, and the first time the school district ever dealt with a fully blind child. I am grateful for all the support we received. They never denied Lauren a single thing she needed. She continued to make academic progress because of it. Though she still had fainting episodes, she seemed to be doing better and better each day.

Very Strange

With so much focus on Lauren, I was surprised when my husband started to push to sell an investment property we owned right before the holidays. It was odd because it wasn't a good time to sell in the market and it was a good investment that made us money. This didn't make sense to me – we had enough going on! He eventually stopped pushing and I just attributed it to him being worried about money.

Then he decided to go skiing out west with Christopher after Christmas. His sister and family were going and had a place with room for them. He felt it was a good opportunity to give Chris some undivided attention. I felt it was an unnecessary expense, and besides that, I would feel extra pressure being left alone to manage Lauren's care. I agreed because I wanted to do my best and make everyone happy.

In the new year, he started teaching for WM again and was traveling one or two times a month. Though I didn't have 24/7 coverage, I did have Carly during the day for Lauren's medical needs and Amanda and Brittany came for some evenings, weekends and an occasional overnight when I needed to get a full night's rest. All in all, things seemed good.

Something very strange was happening though when his travel began. Every single time he went away for a week or longer, Lauren had medical issues that would range from a urinary tract infection to a shunt malfunction that required surgery. I'm not kidding, it really was every single time.

It was hard being the only parent home when it happened. I often wondered why this became a pattern. Maybe Lauren somehow felt abandoned when he traveled or maybe it was coincidence. Either way, I assured her daddy was always coming back. It stopped being a surprise and became something I anticipated: When my husband would leave – Lauren would get sick. Thank God I had my girls around to help.

Waited To Knock, Then Shock

With all his travel, I used to love the nights when my husband was home, and we could do things together and be a family. One night the kids and I were getting ready to watch American Idol. It was one of Lauren's favorite shows and something she could participate in because she could hear the music and then vote for her favorite singer.

My husband was up in his office, and I thought it would be nice if he came down to watch it with us. I went to get him and heard him on the phone, so I waited at the door for a minute to see if it was a business call. What I heard shocked me. He clearly was on a call with a woman, and it was *not* about business.

At first, he denied that there was anything going on and tried to explain away what I heard. It reminded me of his early rehab days when he tried to convince me he had not been drinking and his knee-jerk reaction was to lie to me. It always made me feel like I was going crazy, but there was no explaining away this conversation. He left for a speaking gig early the next morning so we couldn't even have the conversation it deserved until he got home.

When we finally spoke, I confronted him with undeniable proof I found. He finally admitted he'd been talking to this woman for the past year but promised they had not been physical. He cried, saying he felt overwhelmed by everything going on. He said he loved me and our family. He broke things off with her and promised never to speak to her again.

An additional blow was that this woman and her husband were our friends. They'd been at our wedding and spent New Year's Eve with us this past year. I remember the two of them acting very friendly that night, but I brushed it off. How could I have been so blind to what was happening right in front of me? Was I too busy taking care of Lauren to notice or care?

This apparently all started right after Lauren came home from her hospitalization. I was so disappointed and hurt. There was so much going on with Lauren and so much strain on our relationship. Despite evidence to the contrary, I chose to believe they had not been intimate. I told him this type of thing could never happen again.

"You get ONE" I said. This would be the first time my heart would be broken but not the last. We were still going to the hospital in the city for regular checkups for Lauren and her doctor mentioned they had counselors on staff. They told us so many couples experience challenges when they have a child with a serious illness. It can take a huge toll on the family.

Throughout our relationship, I realized my husband held back emotionally. I truly did love him, and I was willing to do whatever I needed to fight for us and our family. We went to counseling for about a year. I had my suspicions that there were issues from his past he wasn't dealing with, but he had to deal with them when he was ready. Things were better though, or so I thought.

Back to School

Lauren was thirteen now and would be in eighth grade in the fall. She regained her strength and was excited to go back to school and see her friends. She hadn't been in school for almost two years. She wasn't fainting as much and didn't need to drink thickened liquids anymore. She was able to walk with assistance and didn't want to use her wheelchair if she didn't have to.

Carly would go to school with Lauren and she would also have a teacher's aide to assist with her special needs. After a few months, there was growing concern about Lauren's ability to focus and keep up with her peers. She was mostly interested in socializing and snacks. By the end of the calendar year, we decided we would try an alternate assessment program so Lauren could focus on mastery of concepts.

"What will it mean for her future if she doesn't get a Regent's Diploma?" I asked the special ed administrator. It didn't matter what the answer was because even the mastery of concepts program turned out to be too much for Lauren. She started developing behavioral issues. She would stomp her foot and smack her hand on her desk. It was Lauren's way of expressing her frustration that she just couldn't keep up. She simply did not have the capacity to communicate how it was making her feel.

We'd been searching for other reasons to explain her behavior, and even had her tested for attention deficit disorder. The educators had hesitated to tell us they thought Lauren just didn't have the capacity for regular schooling. They said they doubted we were ready to consider placing Lauren in any other type of program with all we had been through.

"What we are ready for is to do whatever is best for Lauren!" I said. But maybe there is some truth to what they said. No parent ever wants their child to be labeled or told they can't cut it.

Lauren finished the school year and got to go to her eighth-grade dance. She did not like the loud music but she wore a beautiful dress and hung out with her girlfriends. I went with her and Carly, but after she had her share of snacks and chatting, she was tired. It was time to go home.

On Lauren's eighth grade graduation day she looked so beautiful in her long purple dress with her hair in a ponytail pulled to the side. My mom made her a matching hairpiece out of extra material from her dress. She was very excited to be graduating with her class and wanted to "walk" to receive her diploma instead of being in her wheelchair. Her whole class stood up and gave her a standing ovation as she "walked" up to receive her diploma with Carly assisting her.

Back when Lauren was in the fourth grade with Mrs. H, her class had made Lauren origami cranes during her six-month hospital stay and wished for Lauren to be back at school. There is a Japanese legend that promises anyone who folds a thousand origami cranes will be granted a wish by the gods. Her classmates were so happy that their wish came true and they had their friend not only back in school, but graduating with them.

New Plan

The search began for a new, more appropriate school for Lauren. It didn't sit right with me that we weren't allowed to visit the schools being considered. It was explained the administration would select the one they felt was best. I insisted we be able to visit the schools and see if it was the right environment for Lauren. We finally found a perfect fit at the Brookhaven Learning Center at Samoset. Located within a high school, it was a good mix of kids with varying developmental needs. Lauren would be challenged academically without the pressure regular school offered. She was able to start in the summer program which was only a half-day. She could make new friends and get familiar with the new routine and environment.

Lauren was fourteen now and started ninth grade in a program of academics, practical life skills as well as music and singing. She had Carly with her and a full-time aide and was so much happier. She stopped stomping her feet and smacking the desk. Of course, Lauren would hand out her bracelets to everyone and tell them how she put love, energy and power into every bead, but she also started doing something new. She asked to bring her favorite Werther's candies with her to hand out to everyone she encountered, starting with the bus driver.

"I'm not buying Werther's for everyone in the world!" I would tell her.

Lauren didn't care and she would ask repeatedly until I gave in and let her have a handful. That's my persistent girl, just like me!

Fun Times

With Lauren enjoying her new school and things settling down, we entered another phase of "new normal." More changes came when aides needed to move on with their life and I had to hire new girls. Toni was a new aide and one who brought another level of fun energy into the house and these two would always be laughing. Toni invented something called "the serious game" and the rule was the first one to laugh loses. One of them would always burst out laughing within seconds because of the silly faces or noises the other one made.

Toni liked to draw with Lauren, and I saved many of the pictures and artwork they created. There is one very special drawing they made that hung over her desk. At the time, it was the name of Lauren's website. I chose to use it on the cover and as the title of this book, Lauren's Vision. They also liked to take a lot of selfies of themselves making silly faces or record some of the things they did during their time together. They would proudly show them to me after.

One day Toni said, "Hey Lauren, how about we take selfies with stuff in the kitchen?"

"OK," Lauren said.

Toni then grabbed our stainless-steel tea kettle and held it over Lauren's head. Lauren rolled her eyes up at the kettle with her forehead scrunched and Toni had her mouth wide open with a look of shock and snapped a picture she calls "the appliance selfie." I can't help but smile every time I see this photo and imagine the ridiculous fun they had.

Toni did sleepovers on Tuesday nights. Every Wednesday morning, she would help Lauren get ready for school and she would always say, "Guess what day *IT* is...." That was from the Geico commercial with a camel who went around to everyone in the office asking them to "guess what day it was." It would always crack them both up and became Lauren's favorite day of the week. Lauren would go around all day saying, "Mike, Mike, Mike...guess what day it is!"

Another evening, it was late, and they were having a debate over whether or not they should eat the banana bread that Maritza had made for us. It was Lauren's and Christopher's favorite. Lauren devised a plan on how they could eat it and then blame her brother when asked "Who ate all the banana bread?"

"That's a brilliant idea, my friend. I'm in," Toni replied. These were such priceless moments and soooo Lauren.

Then there was a girls' trip we took to New Jersey to visit her dad during one of his motivational workshops. Toni and her sister Taylor came with me and Lauren. As we took the three-hour drive, we didn't care about traffic and blasted Lauren's favorite music and sang songs at the top of our lungs. When we attended in the audience, Lauren felt like a celebrity when her dad called her up on stage and told her story about challenges she has overcome and how she made bracelets that had become a little business for her. He sold them at the back of the room and people rushed to buy them. He would hand her the mic and ask her to say a few words. It was hard to get the mic back from her. She was a natural on stage and loved the limelight.

Back home, the aides kept her busy with everyday things like visits to Michael's arts and crafts and the Dollar store, where Lauren could roam the aisles and talk to people. On one of our outings, I spotted a group of cheerleaders holding a car wash fundraiser. I asked Lauren and Toni, who were usually up for anything, if they wanted to stop there and meet the girls. "Yes!" Lauren shouted and started bouncing up and down in her seat.

I pulled up and explained Lauren's situation and asked if some of the girls could take turns talking to Lauren while the car was getting washed. The girls surrounded Lauren and listened to her jokes and tips on how their boyfriends should treat them like princesses. The captain of the team asked if they could stay in touch. Lauren was delighted to give out her website. I invited them all to the house one day to just hang out with Lauren and they presented her with a set of pom poms and ribbons for her hair and made her an honorary member of their squad. They invited her to their games as a guest cheerleader. Lauren was so excited to be a part of their team and be "one of the girls."

Torture

At this point of Lauren's journey, it was rare not to have one of the girls in our home at all times to help with her care. Even so, I spent every minute I could with Lauren from the time I woke up until the time I went to sleep. We did lots of fun girl things together like shopping and getting our hair and nails done. Sometimes I needed "adult" girl time for myself.

Her father would usually take advantage of that time to be silly and pull antics that I would never have let occur. One time, I went to visit Maritza, who lived five minutes away. After an hour, I got a phone call from Lauren saying her dad was torturing her and he wrapped her up in cellophane and she couldn't move. I asked her how she got to the phone and she said she hopped over on the chair. I told her I was on my way home and would talk to her dad. When I got there a few minutes later, she was still wrapped up and we both started laughing as she showed me how she bounced over to the phone.

Another time I got home and Lauren told me how her dad put peanut butter on her face and let our dog, Jasper, lick it off of her.

"Ewwww, I would have never let that happen if I was there," I said.

"I know, Mommy and I couldn't believe he did it either and it felt gross when he smeared it on my face, but it was actually kind of fun."

Then there would be the times he tortured us both by intentionally making loud noises in the kitchen with pots and pans or interrupting us every time we tried to say a word. He liked to do this especially when I would go into telling Lauren all the reasons why I love her. He sometimes would stop long enough to say, "Want to know how much I love you? Feel my pinky finger? Now feel the fingernail? Now can you feel the very tip of my fingernail? That's how much I love you!"

She would say "Uh, Oh really!" and came to expect his tortuous silliness and would give it right back to him. Other times he would burp as long as he could just like Will Ferrell did in the movie Elf, which Lauren loved, and would say "Did you hear that?" He taught Lauren to do the same and these were such simple little light-hearted moments that made us all smile and forget about life's challenges

According to Lauren, it was his job to tell jokes and make her belly laugh. She would say all the time, "My dad has three jobs: chiropractor, speaker and to make me laugh." I would remind him that he needs to take the time from all the joking to let her know how much he really loves her. We all needed to hear that.

The Deli-bration

Lauren loved to go food shopping with her dad. Whether they were alone or with one of the girls, they would do something called the "Deli-bration." Lauren would take one of the numbered tickets at the deli counter. Her dad would tell her what number it was. Then, they'd patiently wait for it to be called. When the unsuspecting employee behind the deli counter called out their number, they would both jump up and down and scream and shout as if they had won the lottery.

"Yes, yes, that's us...Oh my gosh, that's us!"

They did this so often the folks behind the counter grew to expect it. They would grin in anticipation and then laugh at Lauren and her dad shouting like two crazy people. Christopher would always be sure to stay far, far away when things like this took place. He didn't like to be the center of attention, unlike his father and sister.

Part of the Family

Emily is another one of those very special aides who came into Lauren's life. She was going to school to become a nurse when I hired her, and she quickly fit in to our family life coming from a big Italian family herself. She was petite, had long dark hair and spoke with a raspy voice. We met Emily through her niece, Taylor, who was one of the cheerleaders from the car wash that adopted Lauren as an honorary member of their squad.

Emily would always jump on the bandwagon to tease Lauren in a good-natured way and joke around. But Lauren especially loved it when Emily took her to visit her family who lived close by. Emily's mom, sisters and nieces all loved Lauren and her philosophies on life. They became extended family and Lauren attended many of their family events including birthdays, barbeques and even got to watch Taylor's cheerleading competition where they won Nationals!

Emily had a keen eye for health issues and was a huge help when my husband was away in helping me monitor Lauren at night when Carly was not around. It was no surprise she would go on to become a pediatric nurse practitioner.

It was friendships like these that added so much depth and quality to Lauren's life. They were all *my girls* that helped me look after and love Lauren and I looked after and loved all of them. These girls will always be a part of my family. I have been to their weddings, held their babies and continue to feel the love of Lauren through them. Life is funny how some people you think will be in your life forever are only there for a short time, and others who you never expected to meet are there for a lifetime.

CHAPTER

Fourteen

Bittersweet Sixteen

Early the following year, Lauren had more trouble than usual walking and complained her right knee hurt. She couldn't put her full weight on it and walked with a limp. She was starting to have accidents as well. Doctors told us that the tumor in the brain can affect various functions of the body and they never knew exactly what was causing her symptoms. This was always frustrating for me that they couldn't explain why something was happening or when it would stop.

She had an emergency MRI just to ensure nothing was changing with the tumor and things looked stable. She also had an X-ray of her knee and all looked fine. But Lauren always displayed physical symptoms before changes appeared in the MRI and I knew to watch her. Over the next several weeks she continued having trouble walking and then she began to drool slightly and had trouble with word retrieval. I knew something wasn't right.

A month after her fifteenth birthday, she had another MRI. It was three months since the last one and showed a thirty percent growth in a small secondary tumor. She went on an oral chemo and we were all relieved she didn't have to go to the hospital every week. The next MRI indicated there was no additional growth and her original tumor seemed to be shrinking. Lauren had a lot of side effects during this time including a high liver count, so her oral chemo dosage was reduced. Still, she was throwing up and had diarrhea, which was causing rashes. She had mouth sores and sties in both eyes. She was physically very uncomfortable, and she started to become very emotional.

Lauren also started becoming fresh with her nurse, aides and teachers at school and it was evident she was having a hard time coping. In addition to everything else Lauren had going on, I decided to have her go back to counseling sessions so she could talk about her feelings. This seemed to really help her. I started going to counseling too to help me deal with the stresses of everything I was dealing with as her mother. It tore me apart to see Lauren upset and having to go through all of this. None of it was fair.

Lowering the chemo dosage seemed to help with her mood swings. She was feeling much better and started getting back to her usual happy self. Unfortunately, she had gained weight and spent more time in the wheelchair than walking. Oral chemo would last much of the year, with all the terrible side effects that came with it. When she finished, we were glad to put it behind us.

College Acceptance

As we rolled into 2014, things were not getting better for Lauren. She was still gaining weight from the oral chemo she was on and having difficulties with balance. We found ourselves in and out of the emergency room to ensure everything was ok. At Lauren's last visit to the doctor, at the end of her oral chemo treatment, she collapsed right there in the office. The doctor didn't think much of it. Lauren had previous problems with syncope (fainting episodes) and the doctor always said to watch for patterns and not overreact to any one thing. It didn't sit well with me, but we were all looking forward to getting on with a chemo-free life and agreed to keep an eye on her.

At the same time, Christopher had a lot of exciting things going on. He was in a badminton championship and would be finishing high school. We were in the midst of taking him to visit colleges. He was thrilled to be accepted at SUNY Geneseo. Lauren was excited, too, because she knew college visits meant meeting other college students!

Summer Celebration or Not

With Lauren turning sixteen and Chris graduating high school, I wanted to do something big for both of them. I decided to throw them a huge two-for-one Sweet Sixteen and High School Graduation Party in the backyard over the summer. I would invite all our family and friends and it would be one big celebration!

It was Memorial Day and Lauren's balance had been off all weekend. As I transferred Lauren from her wheelchair to the bath, I slipped and we both fell. She had gained so much weight, she weighed more than me. She screamed and I was so scared she was seriously hurt. She said her foot hurt. My husband was, of course, away, so I called her doctor and he said to bring her to the ER. It was late at night, but I took the two-hour drive to NYUH.

They took an X-ray of her foot and it was fine. But because of the balance issues, they also took an MRI. It showed her tumor had doubled in size and looked like a large cyst. They wanted to admit her right away.

"No, this can't be! There must be some mistake! She just finished oral chemo a couple of months ago," I said. "Please, get her oncologist and neurosurgeon on the phone!"

They were able to reach her neurosurgeon and he said it might be the result of necrosis, which is a process where, as the tumor dies off, it sometimes creates fluid. I got the okay to take her home, but I had to bring her back the next day for emergency surgery to remove the fluid.

I was able to reach my husband and he got on the very next plane. He flew into JFK and was able to meet me at the hospital. Lauren went through a quick pre-op and then they did the emergency brain surgery. Her surgeon was able to remove fifty percent of the tumor.

The Longest Walk

Lauren was recovering from the surgery. We were again grateful that she did not seem to suffer any complications from this long procedure. My husband and I were sitting in the hospital room with her when I got a call from her oncologist. The biopsy results were in. He asked if we could both come over to his office which was a few blocks from the hospital. Luckily, we had other family members visiting Lauren, so we were both able to go.

When we arrived, we were immediately escorted to the parent consultation room where we waited for her doctor. We were expecting to hear the same news we had previously – that the tumor was classified as a JPA and then we'd discuss what chemo treatment would be helpful to prevent further growth. We sat in the consultation room for what seemed an unusually long time. Dr. A finally came in with a nurse practitioner from the NF1 team. I did not like the look on either of their faces as they sat down and turned toward us. Dr. A paused for a moment before he spoke:

"It's stage four glioblastoma multiforme or GBM, which is malignant. I'm so sorry. There's no treatment for this and unfortunately nothing more we can do."

My world closed in on me at that moment. The room seemed to fade and I was lost in a wave of emotion and disbelief. I was unable to speak or even hear. I could see lips moving and was watching my husband ask questions but nothing registered. I was in complete and utter shock.

Tears welled in my eyes and streamed down my face. My mind wandered all over the place and then reality set in – I was brought back to the room I temporarily floated away from and I could hear voices as I started to focus. What questions do you ask when you get the news your child has a malignant tumor? My heart was in my throat as I began to ask my questions, partially in hysterics:

"What do you mean there is nothing else we can do?" I finally said.

"Can't we call her neurologist and see if he can do another surgery?"

Dr. A just looked at me with a solemn, helpless look I will never forget.

"What about clinical trials? Aren't there any clinical trials or other drugs we can try?" I asked as my husband now sat there in silence. The doctor just looked at me and slowly shook his head.

"I am not throwing the towel in on her," I said with tears rolling down my face.

Dr. A then looked at me with his gentle smile and said:

"Lisa, I have never met a parent who has done as much for a child as you have done for Lauren. I am telling you there is no cure for GBM. It's very aggressive."

"You always told me 'You never know what is around the corner,'" I said to him.

"Please don't throw the towel in on Lauren, not now, not ever!" I pleaded.

"How long?" My husband asked.

"We don't know. Maybe a few weeks to a few months," he replied.

I couldn't believe it. I wouldn't believe there was nothing else left to try. With tears still streaming down my face, we left the doctor's office and began our walk back to the hospital. It was the longest walk of my life. We held hands as we walked in complete silence. We passed a church along the way that we had passed many times before. This time I went in to say a prayer. When I came out, I sat on the stoop outside of the church and put my head in my hands and started to sob uncontrollably.

"This can't be happening," I cried. "Not to our little girl."

Marine Baby Strong

Things felt surreal when we got back to the hospital and shared the news with our family members. I had to be strong for Lauren right now. She had another ten days in the hospital to recover from this major brain surgery. The surgeon had to build a mesh insert with a titanium plate to keep everything in place. Her recovery was first and foremost; she didn't need to know any other details. She just needed to focus on getting her strength back. When she came home her balance was still a little off, but she went back to school. Try to keep things normal we reminded ourselves again – while we figure out what to do next.

While I was contemplating quitting my job so I could spend all remaining time with Lauren, we got a call from the doctor's office. They said there was a chemo drug they thought we could try, Temodar, five days on, three weeks off. I knew they would find something!

"This is not how this story is going to end!" I said to myself.

I would also continue my research on the internet on GBM tumors to see what else might be out there. If there was something out there, I was going to find it

I have said I'm like my dad when things get tough. He would always proudly say he was a Marine, trained to adapt and adjust to any situation. Often times that would be followed by him singing the Marine Hymn, Halls of Montezuma. Marion would always say that makes us Marine babies. So once again, I put on the armor to transform into the warrior to "adapt and adjust" to get things done. I could hear it latching up all over my body preparing for what was yet to come.

Party Is On

Our two-for-one party was two months away. We weren't sure if we should cancel or not, but finally decided the party would go on. We would celebrate all the things we were grateful for and all the possibilities yet to come. The words of Dr. P, the orthopedist, kept coming back to me. I could hear him say "keep things normal, enjoy your life". That is what I was determined to do for my family. I would not let Lauren's grim diagnosis stop us from living our lives and continue hoping for a miracle.

Lauren's lab work looked good and she was starting to get her energy back just in time for her party. She was so happy and looked absolutely beautiful in her hot pink cocktail dress, wearing a tiara over her blonde highlights. Looking at a picture of our family on that day, and the smiles on our faces, you would not know the prognosis that hung over her head.

I got a DJ sound system complete with microphones for music and speeches. Marion helped me decorate and brought plenty of Lauren's favorites like Swedish Fish and M&M's. Trish went all out with a brownie sundae and dessert table that Lauren couldn't wait to have. We had the photo booth Lauren wanted and the dunk tank that Chris requested. It was a gorgeous summer day, and all our friends and family came out to celebrate. Chris would soon be off to college and Lauren was on the new chemo. We all hoped and prayed there would be many more parties yet to come.

LC Tips of the Day

I did my best to stay positive and look for the silver lining in all things. That's why one day I asked Lauren if she had a tip for other people on how to stay happy, positive and healthy, so we could continue to spread her signature HPH philosophy. She loved this idea and I started to record her tips and post them on my Facebook page with Lauren always ending with, "This is LC signing off!" At first, it was just something she and I did together. Then my husband got in on it and before we knew it, everyone she knew was asking her for a tip of the day.

I decided to create a YouTube channel for Lauren and posted many of her tips there. They ranged on topics from simple advice like, "Love Your Family," or "Study Hard," to ones where she cracked herself up, like "Go Big" and "Try New Things." You just had to laugh when she laughed.

One of my favorite tips was a very sweet one called "Live it Up" where she explained her philosophy of living life HPH and then encouraged everyone to drink a pina colada. Another favorite was called "Go With The Flow." I recorded this one while we were sitting in the hospital waiting for MRI results. My husband was asking Lauren about a tip for the day and then he said something to make her laugh really hard. She turned to him and said, "I think I just peed myself." And he turned to me and said, "Sometimes you have to go with the flow." It was hysterical and one of those moments you really just had to laugh or you would cry.

Lauren and her positive outlook on life never ceased to amaze to me. Here are some of the other tips of the day we recorded:

Don't forget to smell the roses,

Expect the unexpected,

Live for today,

Do something crazy,

Go on vacation and live your life,

Exercise is really important,

Have fun,

Eat cake,

Breathe and smell the fresh air,

Blondes have more fun,

Have a safe Halloween,

Don't sweat the small stuff,

Make a decision to be happy,

Get a donut,

Be fashionable,

It's all about the bacon,

Have faith and hope,

Lay out in the sunshine,

Mix it up and Live HPH!"

I was doing all I could to stay positive. Lauren and I did her tips of the day everywhere we went, and I continued to share them online. We took lots of trips that year to her favorite places like Aruba and Florida in hopes of making her happy. All the while continuing to search for what could be the next step closer to a cure.

It was a bittersweet year and we did not know exactly what was ahead of us. Was there limited time with my baby girl? Or could we defy the odds and find something to help Lauren get her miracle?

CHAPTER

Fifteen

Spiritual Healing

In my non-stop effort to look for possibilities, I asked my friend what other healing or spiritual things we could do.

"I want to make sure you understand what is happening here," Maritza said. "I think you are getting conflicted about healing work."

"What do you mean?" I asked.

"Healing brings light. Light does all the work and you do not tell light what to do. Light comes in for the betterment of the human. You place hands, you say your prayers, you collect yourself and you go up to the highest place and ask for the highest good of the human being that is being prayed for – without your own desires."

But I was her mother and of course I desired for Lauren to live a full and happy life, here on earth, with me.

"This is being done in cooperation with medical science, divine intervention and a mother's love. A mother's love brings light from her heart and there is no greater healing than that," Maritza said. It is most powerful!

If loving Lauren from my mother's heart was all she needed to heal, we would have seen her complete healing long ago. I think the part of the message I needed to hear most was the one about removing my own desires and expectations, letting go once the prayers were said.

Freaky Deaky

We continued Lauren's holistic treatment: acupuncture, nutrition supplements and energy healings. I was working with Maritza on what I affectionately called our "freaky deaky" stuff where we did spiritual interventions and spoke to Lauren's soul. The messages we got confirmed we were doing everything that could possibly be done to assist her.

"There has been a petition for an extension..." Maritza told me during one session while connecting to Lauren's spirit. "The petition is being looked upon and things have changed energetically. Things have been shifted regarding her lifeline. The petition was formed by Lauren. More time is required."

"I just want her to be well and feel good," I said.

"When the light comes there is no question as to what light will do," she continued. "The light comes to bring forth all that *is* for this individual. It needs no assistance, no agenda, no desire. It needs nothing."

Of all the things I was willing to do, "nothing" was not one of them.

It Goes On But So Do We

The next MRI included a scan of her brain and spine. We had to see how aggressive this tumor was and could not take any chances. The MRI revealed the tumor was still growing so it was recommended to switch to two different drugs, Avastin and Temozolomide.

Lauren was feeling good, and Chris was about to leave for college, so we decided to go on our annual summer family trip to Aruba with Marion and her family. We played Bingo every afternoon by the pool, and it was always fun when one of the kids won. Julianne got Bingo for the big pot, over $700, and decided to give her card to Lauren so she could go up and claim the big winnings! You never saw a girl happier counting all the money that was won. I have a picture of Julianne, Lauren and her aide Brittnay holding up the cash with the biggest smiles on their faces – the moment was priceless! Julianne made Lauren's day!

Lauren had a great trip. She was her usual friendly self, going around the pool meeting as many people as she could, handing out her bracelets and business cards and chatting. One woman was very spirit filled. After hearing more about Lauren's story, she said she would help pray Lauren through this and together we would all love her through. That brief encounter was very special, and her words stayed with me. We would all pray and love Lauren through this.

When we got home Lauren had another mediport surgery so she could start her new chemo treatments. On the day of chemo, she slept up to sixteen hours. She also took much longer and more frequent naps in the days the followed the treatment. There were other side effects as well. All we could do is make Lauren as comfortable as possible and hope things would improve.

Astonishing Results

We were now doing monthly MRIs and the very next one provided startling news. The tumor showed a reduction of fifty percent. The doctors were astonished. Now they all wanted to know more about what other holistic treatments we were doing because they never got results like this before in such a short time. I wondered if this could be the time Lauren's soul petitioned for and was hopeful it was. The doctors still didn't think any of this was a cure, however.

I can't tell you why she responded the way she did or what it was that actually made the difference. All I know is Lauren had her ups and her downs and she always seemed to have incredible surprises for us. Only, it never lasted for too long before something else crept up to change our joy.

Painfully Honest

I started talking with Lauren about the reality of what was happening. Lauren wanted to know why she had to take medicine that made her feel bad. I did my best to explain to her that she was at a critical point.

"We hope the medicine will stop things from getting worse," I told her. "You need to stay strong and I will do everything I can to help you get through this."

I then said to her softly, "The other option is to stop and be done if it's too much. The other choice may mean to go home to heaven, which isn't a bad choice either."

"But I'll miss you, Mommy," she said.

I put my arms around her. "You won't miss me sweetheart, because you'll be in heaven full of love and light and joy and once in spirit, you will be able to see all! You will be able to see me and all of us that you love here. We are the ones who won't be able to see you and we will all be very sad because we will miss you so much." I couldn't tell her how heartbroken I would actually be as I held my tears back, trying to stay strong for her – searching for the right words to say.

It was a tender moment between us, and I think Lauren understood me. "You and I both need to know that love is always there and love does not leave. Unfortunately, a choice must be made and neither one is easy. I know you are telling me you want to be here, but it's really between your soul and God," I tried to explain to her.

"Well, I want to stay here Mommy," she said.

"So stay strong then Lauren, and we will do everything we can do. You go to the doctor, you get the chemo, we will do energy work and say our prayers and do everything we can to help you stay. But just know that Mommy and Daddy and Chris – and all of your family – love you and we are all doing whatever we can do to help you."

"I know, Mommy," she said.

"We need to listen to you, and you need to listen, too, and do your part. You need to do your physical therapy and take your medicine even though it's hard – and do whatever you can to stay strong. I know it's difficult. We have our faith and that too will keep us strong."

I didn't know what else to do at this point but to be honest with her. At least as honest as I could be. These were things you never think you'd have to say to your sixteen-year-old daughter.

Choose to Stay or Go

Maritza checked in with Lauren's spirit.

"All has been said that needs to be said," she told me. "Of course, the physical child does not want to leave but the question now is if the desire of the body, soul and spirit align? Can they all be well with the choice to stay?"

Maritza began to explain, "Her soul is wandering. It is going around and looking and not really having the emotion that the flesh has. It's just going around and looking and saying there's a choice here. Her soul is absolutely considering staying but knows it would be without having the full physical experience of life."

"But why can't she have a miraculous healing so she can have the full physical experience?" I asked.

Maritza explained that what is being honored here is the choice that was made prior to Lauren's coming to this life. The choice of, "this is the life I will live."

"The beauty about that is it never had a timeline or end date to it," she said.

"What about a miracle of a full physical healing?" I persisted.

"You have already asked, my dear, and now you need to leave it with God. You must live and walk in faith."

Lauren's soul will make a choice and now I must leave it with God. I had to accept it was out of my hands and trust. I knew that to keep asking is to not trust. It is not faith to keep asking. I would continue to struggle with this, but I never lost sight of it.

Other intuitive people told me that when Lauren's spirit felt there was no more quality of life, that is when she would choose to quietly go. I remember a healer telling me years ago that sometimes we complete our healing when we pass.

As a mother I wanted my child to be well and to be happy. I was now growing in my spirituality and knew the soul had a say over these matters as well.

Over the years, all my seeking for Lauren led me to the latest medical options but also opened me up to the world of the unseen. It became a huge part of the journey for me and my daughter. To this day it gives me hope and faith that there is more happening here than meets the eye. I truly believe that we are spiritual beings having a physical experience.

Other Alternatives

I was searching high and low for alternative treatments. I knew doctors weren't always familiar with all the trials so I kept searching for anything that could help. I found a raw nutrition treatment plan that would require Lauren and one parent to be away from home for six weeks. We'd eliminate all sugar and follow their nutritional regimen.

"I don't want to torture Lauren like that, and I don't want to be away from her for six weeks. Lauren is not going," my husband said.

"But it could possibly save her life," I argued. "We are fighting for her life here!" I felt like he lost hope and had given up on her, but I wasn't ready to do that. I would never be ready and would never stop looking.

Then I found a doctor in Texas that had a relatively new treatment with so much promise. They used electrical impulses to change the frequency of GBM tumors and stop it from growing, with good results. I was so excited and felt like this was the treatment plan I was searching for.

I emailed all of Lauren's records and finally got to speak with the doctor running the trial. He said he reviewed the info I sent him, but Lauren's tumor had grown too big to be treated in their trial. "No, no, no, that can't be true," I was screaming on the inside. Please, there must be some way she can participate. I did my best to try to persuade him, knowing that sometimes it is just a matter of how you plead your case. But the answer was a firm no, and I was devastated. This was it. This was the last thing I found that could help save her life and we were too late. How could that be?

CHAPTER

Sixteen

What's Heaven Like

As I was searching for treatment options, my husband suggested that it might be time for us to think about making funeral arrangements in case it should come to that.

"How can you be willing to consider that? That would be giving up on her and I'm not ready to do that," I said. I couldn't believe he would even suggest such a thing.

Baby Girl

I spoke with Lynne, who had come to the hospital so many times to visit and play her healing bowls for Lauren. I wanted to gauge where Lauren's spirit was at, even though Maritza and I talked about this frequently. I guess it sounds like I wanted a second opinion.

Lynne said the message she was getting from Lauren was that while she enjoys living in the present moment, she is also tired and doesn't want to fight anymore.

"It's easier for her not to and she would surrender her body if it came to that. There is a very sophisticated higher-self side of Lauren that feels complete and is ready to go," she said.

I explained to Lynne, "Lauren is so sad lately and she keeps asking me how long she has to go to the hospital for. I told her that we should just focus on how many hospital visits until the next MRI and there are only five more chemo treatments until the next one in December. I asked her if she could do five more and she said yes. I'm sure this is what she is tired of. Along with not feeling good from all of the side effects..."

Lauren had been telling me she felt "blah" all the time and didn't know why. She said she just wanted to feel happy again. She was constantly apologizing for all the things she ever did wrong, and I would tell her she had nothing to be sorry for. It broke my heart to see her like this and every time she apologized it made me feel like she was making her final amends. I prayed and prayed...and would have given anything to take this all away from my baby girl.

"My greatest happiness is for her happiness," I said to Lynne.

"The more Lauren's soul contemplates her own existence, the more she realizes she is okay to go, but she says that her greatest happiness is your happiness too and is very connected to you," Lynne said. "There is the possibility that something extraordinary can occur – but that is up to her."

Celebrity Phone Call

Everyone wanted Lauren to be happy. So when my niece, Julianne, was on a return flight from LA to NY and saw a Disney celebrity at baggage claim wearing thigh-high silver boots, she went right up to her. It was Victoria Justice from *Victorious*, one of Lauren's favorite shows. Lauren watched and loved many of the Disney shows of the day including *Hannah Montana*, *Zoey 101* and *Victorious*. Julianne went right up to Ms. Justice and told her cousin's story and went on to say what a big fan Lauren was.

Julianne asked her if she would be willing to say hi to Lauren and give her a quick call. I was right there when the call came in and Lauren was so excited to speak with her. It was a short call but made her day. Julianne said she gave Victoria the bracelet right off her wrist and told her that her cousin made them and would want her to have one.

"This really means a lot," Victoria said and put it on right away. To me she was another angel that came at the perfect time to bring light and joy into Lauren's life.

No Different

People can be so compassionate and kind-hearted, especially when circumstances take a turn for the worse. Lauren never looked at herself as different and she herself was always kind and compassionate of others. That's what Dani remembers most about Lauren. Dani was one of the last aides I hired to help assist her. She would often take Lauren to local stores to do some shopping and for the opportunity to hand out some bracelets, of course.

"People would react so differently to Lauren" she recounted. One person was so touched when Lauren gifted them with a bracelet. The woman offered Lauren $20, but Lauren refused to accept it.

"No, no, I just want you to have them and give them to your two daughters."

"I just can't take these bracelets from you, you worked so hard on them" the woman said. "Well, you can give me a hug then" Lauren said.

Then there was another woman that Lauren tried to speak to in the store and she just turned her back and ignored Lauren. Dani was a pretty good judge of character and did her best to protect Lauren from people she thought would not be open to engage with her. It always struck her as special that Lauren would never say anything mean or judge anyone for not speaking to her and would say something nice like I hope you have a nice day.

"She seemed to honor people wherever they were," Dani said.

Though Dani only worked with Lauren for a short time and was mostly quiet, she and Lauren got quite close. Dani spent every Sunday with us from 8 am to 8 pm. She confided in me that she really felt like part of our family and was grateful for the entire experience.

"Working with Lauren made me realize how much care goes into taking care of the whole person, and you opened me up to the world of holistic treatments that I would not have learned about in school," she said.

"I don't go to church much myself, but by attending church with you and Lauren, I realize how much faith and spirituality means to a person and just how important that is. It not only increased my awareness about spirit but has also re-opened doors for me about God that I had previously closed."

Dani told me that being with Lauren, inspired her to switch from studying to be a physician assistant (PA) to entering the nursing program at Stony Brook University. She felt PA's don't get to spend as much time with patients as nurses do. She wanted a role where she could potentially get to know a person and help treat every aspect. Working with Lauren in our home helped her understand the impact on the family as well.

"It takes a lot of caring and compassion to care for the whole patient, body, mind and spirit and that's what I learned from Lauren," Dani said. I was so touched that she shared all that with me.

Can't Sleep

I was a little surprised by another conversation Dani had with Lauren. It was a few weeks before Lauren's seventeenth birthday when Lauren wasn't able to sleep.

Dani was sleeping in the guest room (which was right next to Lauren's room) when the familiar knock on the wall came followed by, "Daannnniiii, I can't sleep."

When this happened in the middle of the night, Dani would go in to talk to Lauren for a little bit and see if she could convince her to go back to sleep. Lauren always wanted to talk about boys and would ask Dani a lot of questions about her boyfriend. But on this particular night, she had a different question.

"Dani, what do you think heaven is like?"

"Lauren, heaven is where you come as you are and there is no need to change anything. There are no imperfections and you are perfect as you are," Dani said.

"Do you think I will be able to see when I get to heaven?" Lauren asked.

Dani paused and didn't know what to say for a moment. Then she said, "You will be able to see everything. Everything will be vibrant and you can eat as much candy and chocolate as you want!"

"I learned so much from Lauren," Dani told me. "I learned nothing in your life is ever going to be perfect. It's the attitude you have towards anything that goes wrong that is the direction your life is going to go in. Lauren could be bitter, depressed or even angry, but she isn't. She doesn't live that way. She wanted to go out, go to school, meet people and enjoy the food she loved each and every day – no matter what she was going through. Lauren has gone through the wringer and still comes out compassionate and kind. It is such an honor to work with Lauren and be a part of this family and I hope I always will be."

Thanksgiving at Our House

Normally we alternated holidays between our two families. For Thanksgiving, we either went to my sister Marion's or Mammie and Pop Pop's house in Florida. It was typically difficult to get the whole family together on my husband's side, so it was normally just us and his parents. It was a Cummins holiday this year, I thought under the circumstances it would be nice to host it in our home and ask everyone on the Cummins side to join us.

It was the first time we were all together for this holiday. Lauren was still not feeling well. It was so heartbreaking to see her not her normal, happy self. We were still grateful for all that we had, and it was such a gift for the family to be together. My husband loved to cook and was happy to make the entire Thanksgiving feast. I drank a little too much wine and got all sentimental.

"We should always make time to get together for this holiday!" I shouted. "Family was too important not to do this!" My emotions were starting to get the best of me as Lauren's options seemed to be running out.

Time to Choose

Maritza and I checked in with Lauren's spirit at the end of December and found her sitting by the water, conflicted.

Maritza said, "She is nowhere near her flesh and nowhere near her humanity. I hear her spirit saying: '*I know, I know – I have to choose, I have to pick. I have to deal with the reality that this thing came into my physical body. No, I don't want to choose; I don't want to pick! I'm getting away from all of this.*'"

I didn't like what I was hearing, but Maritza continued, sharing what she heard from Lauren's higher self: "'*Everything is my responsibility now. Choose to stay, choose to go, get the miracle, have the miracle, make sure all is okay and make sure she is a good little girl, go to school, take care of herself, eat the right thing (not the things she wants), eat everything they tell her to and allow herself to be placed in a position to have this thing fill her body.*' It's all her responsibility and her job. She doesn't want the JOB of her life anymore, but she knows she has to evaluate her choices and wants to make a decision."

My heart was breaking as Maritza continued to relay what she heard Lauren's spirit telling her, *"Sure, you want me to take that but it's all an empty shell. Whatever "that" wants to do, it will do, but I don't want any part of that. I'm sick of it."*

I wasn't sure what "that" was and wanted to ask what it all meant but I didn't want to interrupt the flow Maritza was in. I listened intently.

"So, she is just sitting and watching, watching grey water. She's in a negative place, in a bleak, grey, dark sea just watching it go by. She needs somebody to bring her back. Grey consumes you and disengages you from the human that you are. She is in space somewhere and spirit has to travel to that stark place and bring her back to this reality, human earthbound place.

There are four spirits on the other side that will assist to bring her back. Both sides of the bloodline come together to assist her. There is movement of things. There was a spiritual surgery performed and it wasn't so much about removing gunk, it was more about the removal of a barrier, whatever keeps her from achieving a better place and allow healing to come."

I listened, but I was still in my own want and misperception of the way it is. I had my own broken-heartedness to contend with.

"Where is she now and what can I do to help? Is she willing to accept healing to stop the tumor or will it take her? Are we making her spirit miserable while she's here because she needs chemo to stay alive?" I asked.

"There will come a point where the chemo is not allowed anymore," Maritza said. "The chemo will be disconnected and the time is coming. So, there is only a few months of chemo left. She will be disconnected from that "life source," because it is "life source" to her. From then on, I do not see "end" for her, because there is no end, but she is curious about "life after life."

There is a saying in the Bible when the flesh falls the spirit soars. Was Lauren ready to release her flesh and embrace her spirit? Is this why she asked Dani what heaven was like?

My heart leapt, but Maritza spoke to me, "She has chosen life for now, but there is a time to this life, not as you would desire it to be forever. There is a time where she will choose to engage in what happens next, away from human and to be in spirit. She has chosen life but just for a time. It is not what mother would desire. Mother would desire for life to be chosen for 20, 30, 40 or even 50 years. So, she has stamped a date on that for the life she has chosen."

I understood that in spirit we don't look at death the way we do here. Spirit looks at life as a decision, a choice. Whether we decide to go or to stay, both are good. But I was this physical child's mother, and I wanted her to choose to stay here with me and live a full, long life.

About Lauren's journey Maritza said, *"It's been a long time of meandering and Lauren has broken many records, staying beyond what she originally intended. We are not being shown how long. It is her soul's choice and one she is not willing to share at this time."*

193

About her current condition Maritza said, *"At home she is also not sleeping well because 'sleep' has been taken from her. She does not know how much time she has left so she does not want to waste any time sleeping. Many things have been taken from her but many things will be given back to her. The tumor is so aggressive and in such a fragile place if they were to do another surgery, we would be at risk of losing the child. We have done our best to starve the tumor and it is turning into liquid form and is smaller than it was and has lost a lot of its power."*

"I just don't want the tumor to be the limiting factor. I want Lauren to know she has the choice to stay. If we have taken away the tumor's power, maybe there is still time for a good life," I said.

"Thrust love into every particle of her being so that in love all that can happen is light. So say to the tumor you are part of this child and I will love you and I will put my 'heart's love' into you and it will contain it there. It will be 'bewildered' and in that chaos, the light will be created," Maritza said.

Maritza was telling me that with the light we send through our love there is healing and spiritual connection, but most of all there is LOVE. It is a different way of fighting it, it diminishes it with kindness and true love.

"It's really the only weapon we have against these things that come to take away our children – LOVE. The biggest power a mother has, which is the greatest power in creation, is LOVE. And that love never diminishes regardless of what happens," Maritza said.

"The formation of this mass, and anything that comes to destroy rather than create, is something that at one point did not know love

194

and created "negative" energy. It finds a way to attach to these human children that we bring into this reality and the actual war that we have as humans is the war that takes away love – but LOVE will conquer all."

CHAPTER

Seventeen

Still Hopeful

With her soul letting us know there would come a time when she would choose to embrace spirit, I finally agreed with my husband to make some arrangements for her passing but only if we did so for the whole family. It was another surreal moment that I had accepted that the time I had left with my daughter could be shorter than expected. No matter what, I still hoped and prayed this would not be needed for a long time to come for any of us.

I found a beautiful final resting place near the water that was only a few minutes from our house. It was a small cemetery near a church that I always admired as I drove by. It was a small, beautiful white chapel with a steeple that was always lit up at night. I got a feeling of peace just looking at it. There were lots of trees and woods nearby. In the winter, we were told you could see the Long Island Sound, which would be so pretty to look at. We picked a place where the sun would always shine just like my Lauren did in her life.

An odd thing occurred while making plans. I told my husband I wanted to buy plots for all of us, so this was a family thing and not a Lauren thing. That's when he said he didn't want a plot for himself.

"Don't you want your final resting place to be next to your family?"

"No," he said, "I want to be cremated and have my ashes thrown into a volcano in Hawaii."

He never mentioned this to me before and as strange as I thought that was, I let it go.

One More Time

Lauren was feeling very sad in January, and we hoped taking a trip to Aruba would help her feel better. This had become her favorite place to go. We had a timeshare but couldn't find an available week at our favorite resort, which was handicap accessible. I noticed a website that had timeshare rentals at the resort and time we wanted, so I contacted the owner. After sharing why we wanted to rent it, the owner actually gifted us the week and would not accept any money.

I always found that challenging circumstances brings out the best or worst in people and here again was one of those times where we got to witness the goodness of others. We went to Aruba during winter break, so Chris was able to come but it really wasn't a very happy trip for Lauren. Nothing we could do or say, even in Aruba, could cheer her up. She was still on her clinical trial medication, and it just came with so many side effects.

Ask For Blessings

Maritza and I did spiritual interventions and everything we could to invoke healing on Lauren's behalf. I prayed and hoped for some last miracle that could change the course the doctors' said Lauren was on. I remember going down to the beach by my house with Maritza and asked her to invoke blessings on the oral chemo Lauren was taking.

We prayed over the pills asking that they be guided to flow into her bloodstream and give all that she needed to be well. We asked this with the intention that her light may shine within her and that nothing can disturb what is not to be disturbed for the healing of her body and progress of her spirit. This was a practice I learned from Pranic healing to bless our food or in this case, pills, and then let go and let God. I remained so hopeful and continue to do whatever I could. There were plenty of times my faith waivered, but Maritza would always remind me that we walk by faith and not by sight. I needed that encouragement now more than ever.

Coldest Winter Ever

It was a brutal winter on Long Island. We got over fifty inches of snow and February would be the coldest month on record. On days like this, Lauren used to love to wear fuzzy socks and snuggle with me under soft blankets. There was so much going on with her, the last thing I expected was to get a phone call from my mother saying something was wrong with my youngest brother, David.

At the time, David wasn't working and had a falling out with his best friend. He had been isolating himself in his apartment in the basement and she didn't realize the state he was in until one day he came up and just sat on the couch, not saying a word, eyes glazed over. It was the same place my father sat many years ago when he died suddenly of a massive sudden heart attack. My mother was frightened.

She didn't know what to do so she called me. "Lisa, I hate to bother you with all you have going on, but David is not himself and I don't like the way he looks."

"I'll be right there," I told my mom.

I left Lauren in the care of Carly and got to my mom's as fast as I could. As soon as I walked through the door, I saw my mother was right to be concerned. David was in a bad state. I spoke to him softly and told him we needed to go right now, and he packed a bag and came with me. I got him checked into a hospital that was highly recommended for someone going through depression.

My three sisters and other brother all rallied around him. Not only was he suffering from depression, but his drinking had increased and there was a lot of intervention required. After a couple of weeks in the hospital he was feeling better, and we helped him come up with a plan to get his life back on track.

While in the hospital I remember getting him a card with a poem about an oak tree and how he needed to stand strong like the mighty oak. I also gave him some of Lauren's bracelets to give out and he felt like he was helping others who were going through similar circumstances. He said it provided additional encouragement. We filled him with love and support and in turn he was able to provide it to others. Lauren called him to say if she could do it, he could do it! It gave them both purpose. He kept the recording of her call.

David got out of the hospital and attended counseling while living with my sisters Annalise and Cathy in Long Beach. Shortly after, he found a job and life seemed good for him. He got a second opportunity to live his life HPH, and we all did what we could to support him and hoped this would continue.

I was doing what I could to help my brother, but I was beginning to feel exhausted with everything that I had to handle. I could see things were slowing down with Lauren. I tried to talk to my husband about my feelings. He would get an indifferent look on his face, and I could see it was too much for him. How I longed just to be held and told everything was going to be okay.

This was a hard time for both of us, I know. I especially felt disconnected and lonely when he traveled. It was nice to have Carly and the girls to help and talk to, but it wasn't the same as having my partner there with me. He continued to travel for WM and it seemed to dump snow every time he left during this brutal winter. I was reaching my breaking point physically and emotionally. When he returned from one of his trips, Lauren hit me with something I didn't expect.

Wherever You Go, I Go

As I was tucking her into bed one night, she said to me, "Mommy, I feel like my body is dying." I sat close to her and stroked her hair. Holding back tears and as calmly as I could I said to her:

"Why do you feel that way, sweetheart?"

"I don't know, I just do," she said. I thought to myself, somehow this child has an awareness that her body is dying. Could this be her way of preparing us both?

Now I had to keep it together and figure out what to say to my baby girl in case it was nearing time for her to go. So, I held her and kissed her and said to Lauren as softly and sweetly as I could that we can never be sure when it's our time to go. Then I did my best to explain to her what would happen if either one of us got called back home to the other side – to heaven.

"You know how much I love you," I said.

"Yes, Mommy."

"Well, you get to take all that love with you wherever you go."

"Really?"

"Yes. And no matter who goes first, the love goes with you."

I reminded her that everyone, at some point, leaves their physical body and goes back to spirit.

"Always remember, Lauren, wherever you go, I go – and wherever I go, you go."

All this seemed to reassure her. I tried to make things a little lighter by making a pact between us that we would come back in another lifetime with no drama.

"You know Lauren we can come back as sisters or BFFs, and live a great life."

"Promise?" she said.

"Promise" I said.

I went to find my husband and asked him to speak with Lauren. If this was some kind of revelation she was having, I wanted him to have the opportunity to let her know how much he loved her. He sat by her bedside and I let them have some time alone. I came back in and we both reminded her how much we all love her. I fell asleep with my arms wrapped around her.

I never stopped praying and expecting a miracle for her. I hoped that every day could be better than the last, and as her doctor would always say to us, "You never know what's around the corner."

Section Three
P O W E R

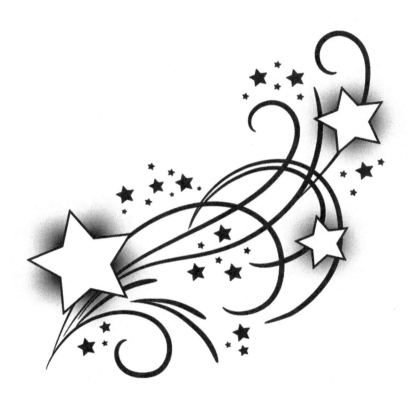

CHAPTER

Eighteen

Not As Planned

Lauren's birthday was coming and she was going to be seventeen. With all the snow we had, we thought it would be great to head south to celebrate. We asked Lauren if she wanted to visit her grandparents in Naples for her birthday and she said "YES!" She always loved to spend time with her Mammie and Pop Pop and loved to be in the sunshine. Lauren was born around Easter and her birthday would be during spring break this year, so Chris could join us. My niece Jessie, who was a school teacher, was also able to come.

A day or two before we left, Lauren said she had a headache. We were concerned because the last time she complained of headaches was when the tumor was discovered. Her doctor prescribed steroids to help reduce any swelling but said it was ok to still go on our trip. She had just finished her oral chemo and the doctor said we would discuss new options when we got back.

So Tired

In Florida, Lauren swam in the pool and sat in the sun as if to embrace all that life had to offer. She liked to float, and we could only imagine how freeing it was for her to be in the water and not feel the restriction of her wheelchair. Lauren was very tired on this trip and taking longer than usual naps. She kept asking how come she was so tired all the time. She knew things were not right.

"Your body knows best what it needs and if it is tired that means it's going into rest and repair," I said.

I was so worried about her and hoped the doctors would find a new chemo with fewer side effects while we were away. I wasn't sure how much longer she or any of us could go on like this, but what I knew for sure is I just wanted more time with my daughter.

On her birthday, we had a party for her in the community room by the pool. My husband was called up to make a speech by his dad, but he could hardly get the words out before breaking down in tears. I asked Lauren if she would like to say a few words and she spoke to everyone who gathered here with the grace and the elegance of a princess, thanking everyone for all their love and support. She ate her cake and asked me to take her back to the room. Before she left, Pop Pop asked her if she had any tips of the day and she said, "Just enjoy the party."

Later that evening the immediate family gathered and we gave her our presents. Chris gave her a beautiful three tier necklace with a star, butterfly and heart – the symbols of love, energy and power. Then we told her we had a special surprise. We normally each got her separate gifts because she liked a lot of presents. But this year we explained, there would only be one gift from mommy and daddy. We put the small wrapped box in her hand.

"It's a brick," her daddy told her. She tore the paper and felt the present.

"You got me my own Siri!" she said with delight. We added all her friends and family to her contacts. She was so excited she could use the voice feature. Her first call on her new iPhone was to her Uncle Frankie.

"Whattt"zzzzz Uuupppp?" he said like always and Lauren laughed.

First Class Flight

It was time for us to head home and Chris back to school. Thoughtfully, my husband used his travel mileage to upgrade Lauren and me to first class on the flight home. It was her first time in first class, and she was thrilled. She especially liked the snacks and drinks and loved it when the flight attendant announced her birthday so the entire plane could wish her a happy seventeenth birthday.

As soon as we got home, Lauren's demeanor changed. She slowed down even more. She continued having trouble sleeping through the night, so my husband and I took turns sleeping with her. I used that time when she couldn't sleep to just talk with her and rest with her in bed. One morning she woke up around 5:30 am and she told me all the reasons why she loved me, which is something we did often.

"You're so nice, sweet, loving, caring....super, super nice, super, super amazing, super, super loving and super d-duper sweet..."

"I love you," I said.

"I love you so much too, Mommy," Lauren said. "And I really did try to sleep."

"I know...You did awesome."

"I love you a bushel and a peck and a hug around the neck," Lauren sang softly.

It was a song I would sing to her just as my mom used to sing it to me.

"Yes, I do. Yes, I do. Yes I do!" I sang back.

"Thank you for everything," she said.

"Thank *you* for everything." I said to her.

"For what?" Lauren asked.

"For being the amazing YOU that you are." I kissed her and kissed her some more.

It seemed impossible to imagine that just two weeks before we'd been in Florida sitting by the pool, swimming and walking around town together. Now she was so weak she could barely stay up the entire day.

When The Daylight Comes

We took Lauren back to New York University Hospital for her first checkup since returning from vacation. It was supposed to be a discussion to determine what the next round of treatment would be. Lauren was lying in a bed in a treatment room too weak to sit while waiting for the doc. After the checkup, we followed Dr. A and the nurse practitioner into the parent consultation room. We sat across from them as we listened to them explain why they felt we should not continue with any more chemo.

"We have tried two different clinical trials this year, and nothing prevents the tumor from growing."

Though I knew Lauren was slowing down, this was not at all what I was expecting to hear. Staying true to form, I could not accept it. I went straight into warrior and problem solving mode.

"Can we meet with her neurosurgeon and ask him to do another surgery?" I asked.

Dr. A chuckled and said my hope and optimism never ceased to amaze him.

"I have never met parents who have done more for their child," he said.

"But the time has come where there is nothing more we can do."

I could see how serious he was, and also saw how weak Lauren was and knew in my heart time was running out.

"How much time do we have with her?" I asked.

He paused. "It won't be much longer, possibly days. I can't believe she's made it this long given her current condition."

My heart sank. I couldn't believe what I was hearing. I felt like I had been drunk with hope, but now felt stone cold sober in the stark reality of what he was saying. Still, I had to keep fighting for her life.

"There has to be something else we can try!" I said. "There has to be!"

But they didn't offer anything else, not that day or in the days to come. In a flash, I remembered when her doctor had said that a brain tumor is the kindest of tumors. There is no pain like with other cancers. The body simply starts shutting down and needs more sleep, until it stops functioning.

"Take her home and love her," he said. "Like you always have."

My faith in God is strong and even at that moment, I had faith that there could be a miracle from God to save her. But I also knew I had to trust that if her life was coming to an end, it was her soul's journey and I had to honor that. I still asked in my heart: Had it really come to this? Nothing else left to do?

I went back into the room where she was lying in bed. I went over to hold her hand with tears rolling down my face. A child life specialist was playing her favorite songs on his guitar, but she barely had the strength to sing with him. Her face was full, and her cheeks were red from the steroids she was on. When they sang *Daylight* by Maroon Five, I could no longer hold it together. The words were just too much to bear, "...and when the daylight comes I'll have to go, but tonight I'm gonna hold you so close."

Waiting for the Sunflowers

I had to check in with Lauren's spirit to see where things stood, though it was now pretty clear. Maritza said Lauren's spirit appeared to be preoccupied with the coming of spring. The part of Lauren that was free of her weakened body was playing in the dirt, trying to get the flowers to come up. She was basking in the beauty of nature and feeling the sun on her face.

"She wants the yellow sunflowers to come up," Maritza said.

"The feeling Lauren gives me is she has to protect her choice."

I was always trying to convince Lauren's soul to stay, and it made her feel conflicted in the past.

"Now I find a light soul, waiting for the spring. She has a spirit of allowance," Maritza said. "Lauren is in anticipation of joy and beauty. She is free of needing to protect herself; she no longer feels manipulated to do anything."

Was my deep longing for her to stay keeping her from doing what she needed to do? Did my wish for her healing feel like manipulation to my precious girl?

"She is detached, free, waiting for her body to enjoy the sunlight, the way her non-physical self already is," Maritza explains.

"She already feels bigger, like there is more to her."

Maritza continues to share what she hears from Lauren's soul.

"All is well Mommy, all is well and all will be well. You tell others not to put me in the ground, but you do the same and you do it with your heart and spirit. You cannot put love into the ground! Am I not love to you?"

Tears are now rolling down my face. I immediately understood that Lauren's soul was speaking about the time when her father wanted to choose a final resting place for her when I felt it was too soon and refused to do so. She was letting me know by my desire to want her physical body here even if her soul was ready to leave, I believed I'd be burying her love. In that moment, I fully understood what she was saying. Love cannot be buried. Love does not diminish when a soul leaves the body. I was choked up that she had to ask me, "Am I not love to you?"

Of course, Lauren was love to me. She was the essence of love. She had been co-creating love with me from the beginning. I poured all the love I ever had into her heart and she loved me in return, fulfilling my soul's need for love too.

Now she was asking me to broaden my heart, and detach and only give her my love, not desperation or despair. She was confirming that love will never leave, it is always with us. Just like the night I told her wherever you go, I go.

Feeling Complete

The love between mother and child is the purest, most unconditional love I have ever felt and unlike any love I have ever known. Now Maritza was telling me that the spiritual work here has been accomplished. I have given unconditional love and taught Lauren she deserved it.

"Lauren has been loved from the moment she was conceived," Maritza said. "She chose to stay to co-create love with you. But now she is complete."

"The human Lauren wants what you want, which is for her to stay," Maritza further explained. "But she wants you to be OK if she chooses to go. There is an option for a full physical healing, but it is not what she wants to participate in now."

"I just want her to make the choice that is right for her! I don't understand why she doesn't choose to have a complete healing," I said in despair with my voice cracking from emotional upset. Now I felt like the one that was being abandoned.

"She doesn't feel she will be taken from you the way you feel she will. You will never be separate. Only the physical body will you miss. You will feel her spirit more than you ever have from her physical," Maritza said. "She sees you sobbing. She connects to your pain and your desire for her to open her eyes and see. But it is not necessary. You are the one who taught her to see with her heart. Lauren feels very much aligned, centered and complete in her knowing of this story."

Can't You See

Maritza knew our story, but clearly she was receiving a message beyond anything she had heard between Lauren and me.

"I did wish she could get her sight back before she leaves, so she can look at me, her dad and her brother with her own eyes, is that possible?" I asked in a final desperate plea.

I didn't ask this just for me. Lauren had wished for her sight back for a long time. I guess I wanted additional validation that healing miracles really do exist, so that I could be assured that all of this metaphysical stuff was real. It's so intangible and a miracle like that would make it feel real to me or at least like I had not been out of my mind.

This is the conflict I struggled with. Maybe I had a warped faith in God. I trusted in faith she would be healed if I did what I was supposed to do. I believed that we are co-creators with God, and I was deeply on that journey. I had an undying faith in the power of prayer and healing, though I knew it doesn't happen every time, that doesn't mean you don't ask for the miracle. So I kept asking for the miracle of Lauren to see again; to be fully healed. What Maritza relayed next from Lauren's soul hit me hard:

"...but Mommy, you do not understand, I CAN see you! It is not needed to have physical sight to see. I do see you; I see you all there with my heart and I see you all here with my vision. I see you all! You taught me to see with my heart and I see it all, no change would occur if the eyes were to open."

I was trying to process what was being said and let this come into my heart when Maritza added a final comment from Lauren:

"I can see you Mommy; can't you see me?"

Now tears were streaming down my face.

"I feel terrible that my baby girl has to ask if I can see her," I said to Maritza.

"Of course I see her and all the beauty she is. I'm just trying to work through my understanding of what faith is! I thought if I stayed in faith and did all the things I did, she would have the miracle of a full physical healing. I know and believe with all my heart that is possible! Again, I just want her to realize what her choices are! Then I can somehow find the strength and wisdom to be okay with whatever decision she makes for her highest good."

It was like I was still negotiating with Lauren's soul. I wanted so badly to fix what was wrong and could not take "no" for an answer, even when it came to spirit world. I had to petition for her life. Maritza could see the conflict on my face. I broke down and sobbed.

"I see you Lauren, I have always seen you!" I said.

"You are and will always be my beautiful baby girl!"

It might sound like I was in denial, but I knew exactly what was going on here. I knew in my heart that her spirit had made the decision that it was time to go. She had seen the light on the other side and she was complete here; full of love. What more could any soul want or need? I just wasn't ready to let her go, and I don't believe any mother would be.

The Real Miracle

I could not help but want my daughter to stay and receive the miracle that would completely restore her health. I knew that contradicted what I heard Maritza saying and that the final decision to go home was made.

"Lauren's physical body is tired and has a right to be tired. It is not happy being unable to move and create freely," Maritza said.

"Was it always her destiny to pass at a young age?" I asked as I tried to understand.

"There is no 'supposed' to happen," she added.

"We are always choosing. Lauren says she knows it is a choice at any time to bask in the light of healing, but she has not looked upon that as the miracle. For her, the real miracle is to go home."

"To pass? So I will lose her," I asked still in somewhat of disbelief.

"You will not lose Lauren," Maritza replied. "Love can never die and after she is gone, you will continue to feel her love."

As a mom, I needed to hear this again and again to reassure me that the love I feel would always be there. I already knew all of this and had told Lauren the same. But at this moment, I couldn't get over or accept that I would not have her here with me, in our loving home, with her family. The life I knew, the story I told myself of how life would be, I would have to give up and I would never be ready.

Easter Blessings

With confirmation from the doctors (and spirit) that there was nothing more we could do, we called our family and friends and told them what was happening. We got Chris on the next plane home from Geneseo. Mammie and Pop Pop also flew up from Florida and stayed with us. By the time everyone arrived, Lauren was sleeping much of the day and night. I had to wake her just to eat and felt hopeful that she was still eating and drinking. Her condition was drastically different from two short weeks ago when we were in Naples celebrating her birthday. She was not speaking much and was using her hands to communicate often. For the brief periods she was awake, she wanted to lie down and rest.

We had Easter at our home with my entire family and Mammie and Pop Pop. I felt blessed that she got up to share this holiday meal surrounded by her cousins and the rest of her family. I told myself it was a sign she was going to be okay and that this was just another huge setback – one that she would surely overcome as she had done so many times before.

Her Uncle Jeff (OG1) bribed her to talk at the dinner table and though she didn't say anything and could barely open her eyes, she slowly extended her hand to reach out for the $10 bill and then she tucked it in her shirt, which made us all laugh. That was our Lauren – still there and being an incredible fighter to stay with us, all with her sense of humor intact!

After dinner, we moved her into the hospital bed in our living room. She somehow mustered up the strength and sat up and felt around inside her beautiful Easter basket as my sister Annalise and I sat next to her. She finally pulled out a chocolate Easter bunny and indicated she wanted a bite.

I was hesitant for fear she would choke but I broke off a small piece and watched her carefully as she enjoyed her Easter chocolate. By around 8 pm she wanted to go to bed so her father and brother, together with my brothers, Eddie and David and her cousin Michael all helped Lauren into her transport chair and lifted her up in it as they carried her upstairs into my bedroom. It would be the very last night we would sleep together there, snuggled together and whispering sweet things to each other.

Squeeze My Hand

The next morning was a beautiful and sunny April day. We decided to sit out on the back deck with Lauren and set her up on a lounge chair in her favorite corner where there was no wind and wrapped in her cozy pink blanket – so happy to feel the warmth of the sun on her face. Trish and Bryan were just two of the many family and friends that came by to see her that day.

She was not talking much but responded by squeezing fingers. Chris spent time sitting next to her holding her hand. It was numbing for all of us to see her like this but especially for him since he had been away at school. He lovingly held his sister's hand and spoke to her softly.

"Do you know how much I love you?" He asked her and she squeezed his hand tight.

"Do you love me?" he asked. And she squeezed his hand even tighter.

My eyes welled with tears watching my two babies.

I Want to Go Home Now

Lauren ate lunch and afterward her dad asked if she would like to go for a walk along with me, Carly and Jasper, our dog. She nodded yes. It was still a little breezy, so I wrapped her up in a funky black-and-white zebra-striped blanket she loved as she sat in her wheelchair. We walked down the path she used to walk with her physical therapist toward the beach near our house.

"How're you doing?" her daddy asked.

"Good," she said quietly and put her thumb up. Then, about halfway down to the beach she said very softly in her weak voice, "I want to go home now."

We turned and headed home in complete silence. That night my husband asked me if it was okay if he slept with Lauren. At 5:30 am he woke me up.

"Lauren didn't sleep well the entire night. She was breathing heavy and panting."

"Why didn't you wake me up sooner?" I said as I jumped out of bed and ran to her.

She was burning with fever.

"Let's take her to the shower to try and bring her fever down!" I said.

I was in a panic. We woke Chris up because we needed his help to get her in her transport chair. We cooled her body down with a lukewarm shower. It was so strange because her body was hot and cold in different places and she was flushed only one side of her face. It was like her body was going haywire and she could not regulate her temperature. I washed her hair and body as I prayed the cooling shower would assist her.

She was arching her back and it was difficult to keep her in the chair, but we were able to shower her and took her to her bedroom. I dried her off and was able to get her in soft white pajamas. We brought her down to the living room and she was resting comfortably in the hospital bed we had set up there.

I called Maritza and Judy to tell them Lauren had fever. Maritza came over right away. Lauren didn't respond to us for the rest of the day. She was also very congested. Judy, who was a nurse practitioner, told us we should continuously turn her from side to side to help her body drain the fluid and prevent her from choking.

We all knew this wasn't a good sign and I kept praying. When Judy came over, I remember my husband pulling her to the side. I knew what he was asking her and could tell from the look on both their faces, the news was not good. Judy recalls, "It was as if the light went out from his eyes," when she confirmed his greatest fear that the time has come for Lauren to make her transition to heaven.

Love You Always

That night we slept as a family in the living room and surrounded Lauren. My husband on the couch, Chris on the recliner and I stayed in the bed with her so I could keep a close eye as well as turn her every hour. I wrapped my arms around her and prayed the entire night. If there was ever a time for a miracle, it was now.

All through the night I whispered to her and told her how much I loved her. I wanted more than anything for her to stay but I knew her soul felt conflicted.

"It's OK if you want to go," I finally said. "I will always love you," "Wherever you go, I go; wherever I go, you go," I whispered as tears rolled down my face and the reality of all that was happening was settling in.

The next morning, she was still in a non-responsive state and we took turns sitting by her side. Maritza came back to the house to pray with me, and Judy said she would come by in the afternoon again to check in on Lauren. Around mid-day, Lauren's cousin, Julianne, called and asked if it was ok to stop by and see Lauren. She only stayed a short while but felt compelled to come see her. She gave her a hug and kiss and when she left Chris said he would stay by her side for a bit. I was in the kitchen when Chris shouted, "Mom, come quick! Lauren's not okay."

I dropped the phone in my hand and shouted for my husband who was upstairs. We both ran to her side.

"Help her! Oh my God, please help her!" I cried as I held her hand.

He tried to use the machine the hospital gave us to clear her throat. She was so congested and was now coughing and struggling to breathe. I kept holding her hand and was in a state of panic and then my husband turned and looked at me with incredible sadness and tears in his eyes as he said, "Lisa, it's not working."

"PLEASE, PLEASE, PLEASE keep trying, you have to help her!" I cried.

Her hand felt cold and mine began to shake.

"Can you please get her a blanket," I said with my voice trembling.

"She needs to be warm."

CHAPTER

Nineteen

My Little Angel

The three of us stood there feeling powerless and watched her face go from pink to blue. I knew in that instant she was no more – at least not in the physical. I had watched my baby take her last breath in this world and it was a surreal moment. Chris held her hand, her dad had his hand on her side and I was stroking her hair.

"It's okay baby – go into the light and be at peace," I prayed as tears streamed down my face.

I began to sob uncontrollably with my body thrown over Lauren's. My beautiful, sweet, loving, kind, amazing girl was no longer here. The unimaginable just happened. There are no words to utter here other than, how could any of this be?

1:11

It was April 8, 2015, a Wednesday; ironically, Lauren's favorite day of the week.

I remember looking up at the clock and the time was exactly 1:11 pm. I had been noticing these numbers a lot over the past year and many times my eyes were drawn to a clock whenever it hit that time. I was told 111 had spiritual meaning. I looked it up and read it represents your guides and angels reaching out with love, support and guidance. Maybe it was Lauren's way of telling us she was in spirit now.

Maritza was standing in the kitchen along with my in-laws as they watched everything happen from afar. I turned to them and asked if they would mind going outside to give us a few minutes so we could spend some time alone as a family with Lauren.

As they waited on the front porch, Judy pulled in the driveway and she told them how she felt compelled to come. She was in the middle of having lunch with a friend and knew she had to leave because she felt Lauren's spirit was pulling away. Judy said she felt like Lauren's soul needed some assistance breaking free from her body and could feel her struggle similar to that of a butterfly emerging from its cocoon. She prayed for Lauren the entire drive over.

Carly arrived shortly after Judy. She began crying when she realized she was too late to say goodbye to her best friend. When they all came back in, Maritza asked if we would like her to share what she saw while Lauren made her transition because it was so beautiful. Everyone was interested in what she saw, most of all me.

"The first thing I saw was Lauren's spirit lift out of her body. She gasped in delight as she looked up and down at her body joyfully moving her arms and legs with her eyes that could see." Maritza looked at me and added, "Your dad's spirit was waiting first in a long line of others to assist her back home; family members from both bloodlines, especially all the great-grandmothers."

It was comforting to hear Maritza's vision of Lauren's joyful spirit and speak of all the family members who greeted her. I had read about this in so many books on how loved ones guide us home when our earthly life is over.

Sacred Preparation

In the hours that followed, the women who were present helped me prepare Lauren's body. One final time, these women who helped me love and care for Lauren got to assist me in what I can only describe as one last beautiful experience with Lauren. Together we washed her hair and body. I anointed her with essential oils and perfume, an ancient tradition that goes back thousands of years. It was a solemn time yet felt so sacred and special as we worked together in collective love.

We continued this ritual by lighting candles and called the men back in to gather around her. We all held hands and I asked Maritza to recite Psalm 23. Judy said a final blessing and a prayer for her soul. Sunday Service at Pathways was typically led by Judy, and she always seemed to know the perfect words to say with her soft, compassionate tone. This occasion would be no different. We all cushioned Lauren with love one last time.

I felt a strange peace and unusual calm as I said goodbye to my beautiful, loving baby girl. Oddly, this was one of the most beautiful and touching experiences of my life. I actually couldn't imagine a more beautiful way to honor Lauren's life in the final hours after she passed with this ceremonial preparation with so many of the women that played such an important role in her journey here.

"Are you ready for me to call the funeral home?" My husband asked. I just nodded.

When they came to take her body, mine started trembling and I broke down in tears. I stayed by her side in these final moments and asked them to please take extra special care of my child. I sobbed and put my hands over my mouth in disbelief as I watched them take her from her home for the very last time.

Family and Friends Gather

The wake was mostly a blur. I'm not sure how I even got dressed. I do remember Trish coming to help me pick out clothes and brought me pink jewelry to wear in honor of my girl. Family, friends and neighbors came from near and far to say their goodbyes. There were pictures and memories of Lauren everywhere and the room was filled with flowers and so much love.

It could only be in the true nature of Lauren's spirit and quirky sense of humor that our favorite priest was not able to come on the last day of the wake to say final prayers. Instead, a last-minute sub was sent, who apparently had very little experience at this sort of thing. He started out saying he would be brief but rambled on and on about things that made no sense for us and it was anything but funny at the time. I turned and looked at my husband several times and rolled my eyes. It was all I could do to prevent myself from standing up and pleading for him to stop.

Just then Judy gracefully stepped up and stepped in. She thanked him for sharing and asked if she could say a few words. She ended up saving this special moment by explaining the meaning of every verse in the "Our Father" prayer and could not have been more beautiful. Lauren surely must have gotten a giggle out of this in heaven and gave us all one last thing that we would later laugh about as we said our goodbyes.

My husband wrote a beautiful eulogy to say at the church, but I wasn't sure I would be able to speak. At the last minute, I decided to share the poem about the Oak Tree from the card I had given my brother David when he was in the hospital just a couple of months earlier. I was glad I was able to share this beautiful poem and somehow got through it without breaking down. As mass came to an end, one of Lauren's best friends from school played the guitar and sweetly sang the medley of Somewhere Over the Rainbow/What a Wonderful World. It was Lucinda Judson, better known to Lauren as Lulu. Lauren and Lulu were friends since elementary school. It could not have been a more wonderful way to end the mass.

Tears rolled down my face as we walked down the aisle behind her and the pallbearers carrying her body out of the church at St. Anthony's where she had attended religious instruction and made her sacraments. I remembered the day she walked down this aisle on her Holy Communion; she wore a beautiful dress made out of satin with matching gloves and the headpiece that I had worn on my wedding day. Now she wore another beautiful white dress, bought for her to wear for her seventeenth birthday, as she was laid to rest.

Outside, droves of cars lined up in the church parking lot behind the limo with the giant pink and purple butterfly made out of carnations that Trish and Dan got her. Bill Murphy, the man we bought our dream home from, was a retired cop and arranged a police escort for us that led us down the streets to our house one final time. I continued to quietly weep as we slowly drove past our house that was covered in pink roses and ribbons. My baby was brought home one final time. We paused in front on our house for a moment, and then made our way to the cemetery by the sea.

How Can It Be

For a very long time I kept asking myself how any of this could be? I wondered how the world could possibly keep spinning without her in it. How could the sun rise and set without my baby girl? Yet day after day, it did. I had another choice to make, to choose to participate or stay in bed and pull the covers over my head. There were many days I'd choose the latter.

I never felt a pain so deep. The waves of emotion continued to take me by surprise. They crashed over me, caught me in their undertow and tossed me until I was utterly exhausted. Just as I thought I would never come out of it, I would break the surface, gasping for air. The storm of sorrow felt like it would never end.

I would wake up in the middle of the night in a panic thinking Lauren needed something. I would have to remind myself *Lauren's not here.* I said this to myself over the course of the entire first year, but as time passed, I heard the tone of the voice in my head go from panic: "Oh my God! Lauren's not here!" to a calm and gentle realization like, "Remember, Lauren's not here."

Apologies

In the early days it didn't take much to trigger my tears. One day Chris broke a jar.

"I'm sorry," he said. I burst into tears remembering all the times over the last several months Lauren had said she was sorry for any time she was mean to me or yelled at me, as if she knew she was leaving and wanted to make amends.

One night I heard Lauren call out to me, asking, "Is that you Mommy?"

I woke up and said, "Yes, it's me!" out loud. I was sad and happy at the same time because though I couldn't see or feel her, I actually heard her voice and I felt like she was able to reach across to me from the other side.

About a week after Lauren passed, my husband and I visited her grave. While we stood there the skies opened up and the rain poured down on us. "This is all the angels in tears, feeling our sorrow today," I said.

The sun peeked out through the clouds later in the day and I knew it was Lauren, letting us know the sun would come out again. We'd just have to wait for it.

Hardest New Normal

After a couple of weeks, Chris headed back to college to finish up his semester. We talked about him taking some time off, but he said he wanted to get back.

"If anything changes, let us know," I said.

After Chris left, my husband thought it would be a good idea if we got away. We stayed at a friend's condo on the beach in Florida. It was nice to have some time away from everything to process what happened. We knew we had to figure out yet another new normal for our family.

To process my feelings, I journaled and decided to do something each month to honor Lauren's memory. The first thing I did was make a tribute video for her, which I posted on Facebook and Lauren's YouTube channel. You can look up "Tribute To Lauren" on youtube.com if you'd like to see it. It has many of the pictures referenced in this book. Facebook actually became a form of therapy for me and allowed me to share my feelings about Lauren in the days and months that followed.

I attended mass at the church by the cemetery for a time. They had a beautiful choir that often brought me to tears. Sometimes I would go to just say a prayer and sit in the pew where Lauren and I often sat. Many times, I would be hit by uncontrollable sobbing and would have to leave. I would go and sit on the beautiful stone bench we got to match her headstone that was inscribed with Lauren's Vision and Love, Energy and Power and continue to weep there.

My husband seemed indifferent to all of it: going to church, the symbolic gifts, the honoring of holiday traditions and memorial services by the hospital. If I asked him to come with me somewhere he would, but he was never overly interested. I just figured we were grieving differently. I expressed my feelings outwardly and he handled his inwardly.

In May, Carly and the girls chipped in to buy a weeping cherry tree and we planted it in front of the house. I held a ceremony with the girls, and my family – and we lit candles for Lauren to remind us all what a shining light she was in the world. I planted pink flowers all around and put up butterflies and angel statues. I asked my husband to carve Lauren's initials into the tree and he made a big LC on the side facing our home.

Honorary Diploma

Lauren's classmates and friends were getting ready to graduate high school in 2016. It was Spirit Week at school, and they painted a giant mural in the main hall at the high school to honor Lauren that included her "Live HPH" motto. We were given an honorary cap and gown for Lauren and an invitation to attend graduation day in June. I decorated Lauren's cap with a beautiful script "LC" made out of rhinestones that glittered and shined the way she did. My sister, nieces and I all made bracelets and got permission to hand them out to the graduating class.

On the day of graduation, my husband and I received a diploma on Lauren's behalf. The entire class stood and held up their arms. Each one was wearing the bracelet they received that shimmered with love, energy and power. We didn't realize that was happening.

"Turn around," the principal told us.

I looked out at the sea of faces with arms raised in the air. I put my hand on my heart in gratitude as my eyes filled with tears. Then, I raised my arm in the air and held it there all the way on the walk back to my seat. Lauren's bracelet on my wrist glittered in the sun. There was not a dry eye on the field where the ceremony took

233

place. There was no denying the Love, Energy and Power felt on this special day. I could certainly feel the spirit of my little angel who was surely smiling as she looked down from heaven.

CHAPTER

Twenty

First Year Without Lauren

Regardless of all the honorary events and rituals, it was an excruciating painful and difficult year. I had gained weight and with heavy sadness overshadowing my face, I didn't recognize the woman I saw in the mirror. I felt paralyzed – no longer who I once was and unable to make changes.

I didn't want to get out of bed in the morning and struggled spiritually, especially with the question, "Why?" Nothing felt right, but the one thing I did feel like doing was visiting Lauren at the cemetery and taking care of her final resting place. I left her notes, poems and fresh flowers and decorated her grave for holidays and special events. I never understood before why people did this, but I got it now. It was somehow comforting to mother the sacred ground where my child was laid to rest.

I attended various grief support groups in search of some means to lessen the pain. Though Chris and my husband didn't want to go to grief support or any kind of therapy I spoke with someone every week and found it helpful. I was without Lauren, my husband was detached or traveling, and Chris was back up at school. I felt so alone and had a lot of despair and even some anger that I had to let go of. I found little solace in my meditation practice and was doing the best I could.

Dark Night of the Soul

Six months after Lauren died, I would still burst out sobbing unexpectedly. One day, I was making a cup of tea after dinner when I felt the wave of grief come and crash over me. My husband was sitting in the living room on the recliner with his head in his laptop. I was so desperately sad and needed the support of my husband yet all he did was look up.

"You okay?" he asked.

No hugs, no holding me and no comforting me and telling me it would all be okay.

"Would you come up to bed with me?" I asked.

"I have work to do, but I'll be up soon," he said.

I went into Lauren's bedroom and cried myself to sleep. I woke up about an hour later with no husband by my side. I found him watching television in the basement.

"I just couldn't sleep," he said.

"I must be accustomed to West Coast time since I travel there so much."

This would be the way things would go for the rest of the year. I felt like I was grieving my little girl alone and unloved. I wondered where my marriage could go from here or how long I could sustain it. My husband was emotionally distant, and I felt disconnected from him, which reminded me once more of how I felt after he stopped drinking when we first got married.

I had heard that a high percentage of marriages do not survive the death of a child and never thought that could be us. I also read the first year after a child passes is the toughest and you shouldn't make any major decisions during that time, so I held fast. I was feeling like my marriage was lost but we had endured so much together already. I was sure this would be just another thing we would get through. I decided we each needed time to process our loss in our own way and I should give us more time. My husband's detachment made me wonder, though, what our future would be like or if we even had one.

For me, I was not only dealing with the loss of Lauren but also the loss of my faith. When Lauren left, it popped a bubble in my belief system and in my faith. There were times I didn't know what to do. I felt empty, unmotivated and lacking purpose. I was experiencing the dark night of the soul; everything I thought I believed in and trusted appeared to have failed me. I felt stuck and could barely lift my feet out of the mud. My back hurt and head spun. My only choice was to sit with all of this darkness and despair until I could somehow make sense of it all. But I was doing it alone.

Firsts

They say the "first of everything" after someone you love is gone is the hardest: the first birthday, holidays, family trip, and the first anniversary of their passing. Preparing for Thanksgiving and Christmas were the absolute toughest. On Thanksgiving, I brought out turkeys Lauren had made out of yarn and set a place for her at the table in Marion and Jeff's dining room with her picture and a candle. I bought mugs and markers for the kids to draw stars, butterflies and hearts on as an arts and crafts activity that Lauren would have loved to do. I always liked to go around the table and have everyone say what they were most thankful for. In trying to stay positive, I said the thing I was most grateful for was for having Lauren in our life and all the love she brought into the world.

At Christmas, we put up pink lights on the house and on a tree on the porch with the same pink lights. Instead of gifts from the family I asked for beautiful ornaments for Lauren's tree. Some were handmade and others were store-bought and included angels, or donuts, or something else that Lauren loved. Marion bought plastic globes that we could insert notes, or pictures or other items and "the girls" (who helped me take care of Lauren) all came over for a special Christmas dinner to help make these ornaments for her tree. Putting up the pink lights and her tree with all the special ornaments is now a tradition that Christopher especially loves.

Eighteenth Birthday

For Lauren's eighteenth birthday, I invited all of "the girls" and Lauren's friends from school to come to the house to celebrate. I wasn't really sure if they would want to come and may have thought it strange, but they were all overjoyed to come together for this occasion. They helped me make cupcakes and bracelets and put together a very special collage in honor of Lauren's eighteenth birthday. Dinner featured Lauren's beloved macaroni and cheese and all her other favorites. Lauren's art teacher, Mrs. V, presented us with a beautiful portrait of Lauren she had been working on all year that now hangs in my living room above where Lauren used to sit.

The night before we were all up until midnight talking about Lauren and preparing for the celebration. I noticed how brightly the moon was shining and I went out to wish Lauren a Happy Birthday before going up to bed. I took a couple of pictures of the moon and posted one on Facebook. The next day when I looked at the picture, I could not believe that I could actually see Lauren's face and hair as clear as anything looking down and smiling. It would be another validation for me that my girl was right there with me wherever I go!

Volunteer at GKTW

As another tribute to Lauren, we decided to volunteer for a week at Give Kids the World (GKTW) to give back to other families for all the kindness people had shown to us. We did this in March, her birthday month, over Spring break. Chris loved the experience of giving and said it's the first time in a long time he felt happy in his heart. There were lots of different volunteer stations. You got assigned to a shift wherever they needed help, which could be in the kitchen, restaurant, special events or to be in charge of the rides (which was the most fun). Christopher's favorite was operating the train, the JJ Express, that went around the village.

On one of the days, we unexpectedly ran into a group of volunteers that were from his university, Geneseo. He didn't know that his college ran a program to volunteer at GKTW during spring break. He was excited to see a few of his friends and would look into volunteering the following year through his school. At the end of our trip, we purchased a "memory brick" that would have Lauren's name and birthday engraved and would be used on one of the walkways at GKTW. They keep a map of all the bricks so you can find it when you go back and visit. We've been back many times to see her star in the castle and memory brick.

One Year Gone

For the one-year anniversary of Lauren's passing, our families and friends came for a special mass held at the little white chapel by the cemetery and we all gathered at the grave afterward to light candles and say prayers. It was hard to believe a year had gone by without this precious little one here with us.

Privately, Maritza was able to convey messages from Lauren that were very comforting.

"Lauren wants you to know you came together in this life to assist each other. In a time before you both came to be here, you promised her you would help her free herself from the darkness she thought she would carry for the rest of eternity. And you promised to be relentless until it was done. In turn, Lauren would rid you of your despair from all that you thought you had lost."

There is a spiritual purpose to life, that I believe. What I had to accept was that the deal I had with Lauren was not to *save* her life.

It was about healing her and setting her soul free, not fixing her so she could stay here.

Maritza explained, "Her soul felt complete and that is why she felt she should go." Then she shared more messages from Lauren:

"Love will always connect my heart to your heart, Mommy. Thank you for teaching me how to be strong and for surrounding me with so much unconditional love."

Maritza said our experience together convinced Lauren that she was worthy of love and taught her how to love herself. She could feel all the love and joy and freedom that awaited her on the other side and was ready to go back home and experience that without the constraints her physical body imposed upon her.

"Love is never ending, love is for eternity and my love will always, always be with you, Mommy. I love you. Wherever you go, I go."

I couldn't believe the words Maritza was sharing with me. Lauren was telling me what I had told her. Now I was the one who needed to be reminded.

This did help me put some of the pieces together in understanding WHY. As comforting as the messages were, my daughter was still no longer here physically. It doesn't matter how spiritually evolved you are. There is still such a gap, hole or something incredibly huge that is missing and cannot be filled. I had to learn how to live my life with this immeasurable pain and somehow figure out a way not to let it consume me. But how?

CHAPTER

Twenty One

Broken Glass

After Lauren died, I didn't know what "happy" was anymore, but I hoped in the second year after her passing, I would be able to make progress towards that. My sister, Annalise, asked me to go to a spa and retreat center with her out west. We both thought it would do me some good and we made plans to go to beautiful Miraval Spa in Arizona in June. I had done so much grief work and was starting to get a handle on my life. I wanted to keep things going and thought this could be just thing to help push me forward.

At the same time, I had noticed that my husband seemed to be keeping to himself more and more and seemed very sad all the time. I found him critical, judgmental and very short with me. I thought he might be depressed. He had never sought any therapy and didn't have many friends to talk to, so I was worried.

Grief Sobering Moment

A few weeks before my trip, he snapped at me and said another one of his mean comments.

"Strands of your hair are everywhere," he said, holding one up and looking disgusted. I actually chuckled for a minute and thought he was kidding.

"Is everything okay with you?" I asked. "You really have to stop with this nastiness and talk to me or someone about whatever is going on with you."

"I'm not happy," he said.

Genuinely concerned, I said: "What do you mean, you're not happy? Not happy and sad because of Lauren or not and happy and sad with us?"

"I don't know," he answered.

That was a "grief sobering" moment for me. It completely slapped me out of my grieving and put me into worry about my marriage *again*. Just when I had started to feel a little better and was going to start doing things for myself to try and discover who I was without Lauren, he reveals this news. I was worried about him and our future together. I was also a little angry at him for not dealing with his grief sooner and now interrupting mine. He never wanted to talk about his feelings and was gone so much we barely had time to connect before he was gone again. He stayed up late and didn't come to bed until hours after me.

He said he wanted to "talk" to someone now and wanted to go alone to try and figure some things out. I left for my trip worried and confused. I didn't know what I would be coming home to.

Time to Reflect

Miraval was just what I needed to gain perspective on my life and was so good for my soul. I wished I could have used the time to focus solely on me without the worry of what was going on with my marriage. Regardless, I made some wonderful connections and was able to take some healing workshops. I took a class on sound healing using Tibetan bowls and bought one to bring home for my own healing practice. I met with a social worker and discussed what was happening at home. She gave me advice I continue to use to this day.

"We are all 100% responsible for 50% of a relationship. Each person is responsible for their side of the equation. If and when you don't get a response or connection back in the way you want, you have a choice to keep doing your side of the equation until you decide not to anymore."

I realized that I had given everything I had to my family, including my marriage. My family was the most important thing to me, and I was always giving 150% and was relentless in trying to fix whatever was broken. I also realized that I needed to take care of me and do my part and let my husband do his part. He needed to start showing evidence that he wanted this marriage to work and to move forward together.

I realized all the years with Lauren put us in responsive mode and focused on her. Now we have come to a fork in the road and we

245

both had choices to make. The counselor encouraged me to get clear about who I am and what makes me thrive as a person. I spent my entire life taking care of others and putting their needs first. Now was time for me to figure out my authentic self. She reminded me I don't have to wait until I'm not sad anymore, and I don't have to wait for my husband to make a decision. I could choose to invest in my own well-being and happiness.

I hated being thrust back into uncertainty and fear. I had spent the last year finally being able to rest from being on high alert all the time with Lauren and now I could not trust what my husband's intentions were for our future. I went home feeling cautiously optimistic. I wanted my marriage to work and was willing to put in the effort it deserved, but I wasn't sure my husband was willing to do the same. Looking back, he had never put effort into our relationship or anything else, especially once something got hard. He called it being "recreationally inclined."

First Solo Event

While all of this was going on with our relationship, my husband was planning his first big solo training event in Las Vegas. I helped him with every detail and had every intention of being there to support him. Then he dropped the bomb that he didn't want me or Christopher there. It didn't add up. Looking back, I realize this was a clear signpost that something was really off and not just delayed grieving. But he was very convincing at the time.

"This is the first thing I'm doing on my own and I don't want to share the moment," he tried to explain.

"What the hell?" I said confused and hurt.

Maybe he still just needed some time to figure things out, I thought. So, I continued to help him, and he had a successful event in that at least we broke even. Afterward, he wanted to buy himself a very expensive watch to commemorate the event. Once again, this was money we didn't have, but he really wanted it and wasn't really asking me...and I was not about to say no to anything that would cause more tension between us.

Other Trouble

About a month into his junior year, Chris did not sound good to me. After asking a lot of questions one night, he finally admitted things were not going well and he was not himself. He had stopped going to classes and didn't see the reason or meaning to things anymore. He had been having trouble in his relationship and had recently broken up with his girlfriend of three plus years. I told him we were coming up right away. When I spoke to my husband, he said there was no need for both of us to go and he would take the ride alone.

"There is no way I'm not going up there to see my son. If you don't want to come, that's fine. But I'm going."

We both went and found out Chris wasn't feeling himself for almost a month. He admitted he was skipping classes, partying and playing video games instead of focusing on his school work. Nothing seemed to matter to him. He seemed to be depressed and admitted the loss of Lauren was finally hitting him. I contacted his dean to discuss what kind of support we could set up. The dean then reached out to all of Christopher's teachers as well as the campus counselor and things were put in motion to get him support. It seemed my husband and Christopher both had delayed responses to losing Lauren and it was now catching up with them.

Marriage Intensive

Things were not getting any better between me and my husband. He barely saw his therapist between all his traveling and did not want to talk much about it with me. I reached a point where I said we needed to do something intensive to get things back on track with us or we would need to figure out next steps. I was not willing to keep living like this, walking on eggshells with him. I could no longer pretend that everything was okay between us, especially in front of Chris. To my surprise, he agreed to a marriage intensive.

Her Jag

During this time, my husband talked me into selling my Jaguar because it was getting old and needed more and more work. It had sentimental value because Lauren loved that car and she always called it "her Jag." When she was young, she asked if it could be her car one day. Even after she lost her vision, she would say, "When I get my vision back, I want to drive the Jag."

My husband took me to an Infinity dealership and had them show us the latest model with all the bells and whistles. I would have been happy with a pre-certified car and spend less money. It was not exactly the car I would have wanted for myself, but *he* loved it and said this was the one *we* wanted. I agreed because I thought it was time to explore and let go of some my attachments to things of the past and start new beginnings. If he was willing to buy a car together, I thought that was a sign he was investing in our future.

Faces of the Heart

I did all the research and found three solid options for different types of intensive marital counseling. We agreed on a three-day marriage intensive that required us to fly out of state to see a wonderful woman named Debbie who was both patient and kind and had lost a child of her own. I found the counseling tremendously helpful and, though expensive, I thought it was worth every penny if it could save our marriage and help us get a new start. This is one time I didn't care how much something cost.

At the end of the intensive, I still did not know which way things were going. It was decision time. I was clear from the start that I was all in, but I wasn't sure what my husband's decision would be. At the end of the third day, he said he was all in too. Honestly, I was shocked – but happy. She had us perform a ceremony on the beach where we promised each other to let go of hurts of the past and focus on our future together. It was really beautiful and meaningful.

We would continue to have follow-up sessions with this therapist individually and together. We would need continued support to form some new habits and a healthy relationship. I breathed a sigh of relief but knew we weren't out of the woods just yet. It would take work and behaviors would have to change. Time would tell.

Mt. Kili Climb

Chris came home for Christmas break and said while he was feeling a little better, he was still not himself. He was really happy with the counselor he was seeing up at school and even agreed to see someone while he was home. I took him to see a doctor while he was home for a physical and he went on a low dose of medication to help with his depression.

Out of the blue, my husband announced he wanted to go to Africa to climb Mt. Kilimanjaro.

"Are you in or out?" he asked me.

"What? When?"

"Chris and I are going to Africa to climb Kili in January."

"Well, if you're both going, I'm going too!"

This was not on my bucket list by any means, but I looked at it as an exciting adventure with my husband and son that would metaphorically help us all "rise up" and have a new beginning.

I was a little concerned about the cost since he spoke about flying first class along with private guided tours for climbing Kilimanjaro and Safari.

"Let's consider traveling coach," I suggested.

"Well, you can fly coach but I'm going first class," he replied in a snarky tone.

He was always quick to spend money we didn't have and, in order to feel safe, I needed to have a cushion, or a "moat" as he liked to call it. When I asked how we were going to pay for a trip like this, he said he had a gig coming up that he would pay for the whole thing

"And if something happens to that gig?" I asked.

"I'll find a way," he said. (Spoiler alert: His gig was canceled.)

I wish I could tell you that climbing a mountain and undergoing every change of climate in the weather and watching amazing African sunrises and sunsets was enough to reignite our relationship, but it was not. Each day he said or did something to confirm my sense that he was pulling away. All he seemed to care about was having pictures taken of himself at every milestone of the trip.

I brought a picture of Lauren to keep my promise of everywhere I go she goes, and we took a family picture with me holding her picture and a bracelet at the top of the mountain. I had brought Lauren's bracelets for our guide leader, Ellie, and the rest of the team on our private climb. I spoke to Ellie about Lauren, and he said he could feel the love we had as a family and we were very lucky.

My husband got mad at me a couple of times when I could not keep pace especially when we were getting close to the peak right before sunrise. I told them to go ahead and I would be right behind them.

"No, mom we climb as a family," Chris said.

But my husband said, "C'mon Chris, we'll meet mom up there," and left me behind as he made his way to the top of the mountain.

This was supposed to be a magical trip for us, and it was anything but. He complained to me that he had a hard time staying in the same two-man tent because my stuff was everywhere. We had all of our belongings for a two-week trip in a backpack. His stuff was just as spread out as mine and it was just another indication of where he was at. He also got mad at me when I had to take bathroom breaks and would need a minute to rest after climbing to a secluded space.

"Pole, pole (pronounced po-ley po-ley)," Ellie, our guide would keep telling us. That's Swahili for "slowly, slowly," and would be the way we'd get to the top. This trip taught me patience, and I knew I could do anything if I just kept putting one foot in front of the other. It was going to be the same with my marriage. I was going to keep walking in the direction I wanted to head and would ultimately get there, or so I hoped.

Back to GKTW

Chris was feeling better and better after our trip. He went back to school excited to share stories from his trip to Tanzania and the Serengeti. Not only did he get to see every African animal in their natural habitat that you could possibly want to see, but he also obtained bragging rights for making it to the top of the mountain. It was such an amazing thing to do as a family, and Lauren was right there with us in spirit and in the pictures we took along the way.

Chris looked into his school's annual GKTW trip and really wanted to return and volunteer again because of how happy it made him to help other families in similar situations. There is just something so special about being there and how good it made his heart feel. He put in for trip leader and was selected! When he got back, he not only talked about what a great experience it was but how he would love to work there after he graduated. I was grateful he had such an amazing experience and was turning a corner in his life. I hoped the same would happen with me and my husband.

Mother's Day Surprise

The day before Chris was to come home from his junior year at college, my husband made me a really nice dinner, lit a candle, opened a bottle of my favorite red wine and poured me a glass. I was excited to see he did this and thought he was finally starting to come around. After dinner he said he wanted to talk and I knew it was going to be really good or really bad.

"I've decided to leave," he said.

It was another one of those surreal moments that took me a little bit to fully grasp what he just said. Then I realized he spoke what I already knew in my heart must happen. While I was deeply saddened by this truth, somehow I managed to stay perfectly calm, took a deep breath and said:

"Ok, I agree, it's time for us to separate since things aren't getting better between us. Maybe some time apart would do us both some good."

And then he dropped the next bomb that I was not quite ready for:

"I plan to move to Vegas," he said.

"Why would you go to Vegas?" I asked dumbfounded.

"The West Coast is where I do most of my business and Vegas is where I want to be."

"How can you move that far from Chris?" I pointedly asked and was surprised by his answer. "He needs both of us now more than ever."

"Chris will be fine with you. This is something I have to do."

WTF! Is he serious? Everything was happening so fast, my emotions swirling...I knew we needed some time apart to figure things out between us; I just couldn't for the life of me understand why he wanted to be so far away and remove himself from *everyone's* life.

We went from working on our marriage to, "I'm outta here." When we spoke to our marriage counselor (yes, we were still in marriage counseling), she suggested we create an informal separation agreement based on what we both wanted and expected during our time apart. The next hard part would be telling Christopher.

Chris came home the next day so happy, feeling much better and looking forward to being home for the summer. We waited until he was settled in, and I made him one of his favorite meals like I always did when he came home, and then sat him down in the living room and broke the news to him. "Things haven't been going well between me and your father for some time now," I said. "Your dad and I have decided to take some time apart...We're sorry you have to find out on your first night home, but thought it was important for you to know." Chris just looked at us with tears welling up in his eyes and said he understood. He shared that he wasn't completely surprised and had seen the writing on the wall.

He wanted to spend some time by himself to process the news and went up to his room. Christopher's father and I took turns to talk to him individually. He didn't really want to talk much to either of us. When I sat with him, I tried to explain that we really did try to work things out and was sorry for having to keep secrets from him. I promised him, especially with Lauren, that we would always be honest. At the end of my talk, I hugged him and told him no matter what happened, we would always be a family.

Even though I knew separating was the right thing for us at the time, I was still concerned about the distance. I keep telling myself this would be good for us and somehow rediscover ourselves and in the end, come out closer and stronger together. Nothing seemed to make sense, but what he said next would explain everything.

From Hero to Zero

We each spoke to our marital counselor individually about what we wanted during our time apart. She had given us a template to follow to create an informal agreement and said we should discuss it with each other. As I went through it, there was one very specific question that needed to be answered. Did we want to agree to not see other people during the separation? I knew my answer was yes, but wasn't sure what his answer would be?

"No, I won't agree to that," my husband immediately retorted when asked.

"Why not?" I asked as I turned and looked at him with heightened anxiety. He quickly responded, "I already know who I want to see."

Now I had more questions. As I pushed him, he finally admitted that he had been having an affair with a woman for the last several months.

"While we were in marriage counseling?" I asked.

"Yes," he said.

"How could you possibly work on our marriage while having an affair?" I said.

"You wouldn't understand" he said.

He was right I couldn't understand.

"Were there others?" I asked as I held my breath, never expecting to hear what he had to say next.

He looked at me unapologetically and started telling me of all his past infidelities and unscrupulous behavior. From what he was now telling me, he had made a mockery of our marriage and there was nothing but lies and betrayals for the last six years, maybe longer. I know statistics are high on many marriages ending after the loss of a child and never thought we would be one of them. But what he told me had nothing to do with the loss of Lauren because this had been going on for years.

"Stop, that's enough," I said when I couldn't bear to hear any more.

"Why are you telling me of all this now?" I asked.

His explanation floored me.

"Because I want to live a life of integrity and tell the truth."

INTEGRITY! That word swirled in my mind. He just told me everything in our life for the last six years has been a lie. How could he possibly use the word integrity to describe the way he was acting now? My head was spinning, and I felt like I was in another living nightmare,

"How could my eyes have been closed all this time?"

It was time to live my life with my eyes wide open and it felt surreal. As all of this settled in and I got more clarity, memories came flooding back from the past and started to make sense – all his traveling "to build his new career" leaving me to handle everything without care, departing so quickly after the break-in, the affair after Lauren came home from her six-month hospital stay, his desire to sell our investment property when the market was bad, his pattern of staying up late and not coming to bed with me, not wanting me or Chris at his events, his refusal to have his final resting place with the family, climbing to the top of the mountain without me at Warrior camp and Mt. Kili and so much more. He even stopped wearing his wedding ring but said it was because he fingers were swollen on stage and he didn't want to lose it and I believed him!

It finally dawned on me that he had checked out of our marriage many, many years ago, living a double life the minute he walked out the door and into the limo in his fancy suit and expensive watch. He stepped out of our house living one life and on to the "stage" living another, leaving his family and everything else behind him. My head was reeling from all his empty promises...how everything he was doing was for the family, yet in the end it was never about us. It was like he transformed into a totally different person and created a fantasy life where he had people adoring him and running to accommodate his every need. Now I could see he was only interested in what made him feel good – at any cost – fooling everyone, most of all me.

On that day he went from a hero to a zero. He left a few days later to go to Vegas and find an apartment. He came home and said he found a place and it would be ready in four weeks. So, he packed up a pod with his clothes and left so much behind. He arranged to have his car shipped and took an early morning flight right after Father's Day with seemingly no remorse and no regret. He had become a complete and total stranger. He finally took off his mask and showed me who he was, and I had no choice (as Mayo Angelou would say) but to believe him.

Now I needed to figure out what normal looked like for me and Chris and somehow ensure we would both be okay without his sister and without his dad. Chris surprised me with his compassion and wisdom. When I asked him how he felt about his dad, he told me about a broken glass. "Mom, you know when you drop a glass on the floor, and it breaks into a million pieces? You can try and pick them up and put them back together but no matter what you do it will never be the same."

CHAPTER

Twenty Two

Stronger Than You Know

O nce again, I had to put the armor on and convince myself I could get through the unbearable. The world as I knew it was changing once more, but my biggest concern wasn't for me, it was for my son. He experienced so many losses at such a young age. I honestly didn't know how either of us would get through another life-altering event. Not to mention that this changed everything that I thought I knew, believed and trusted about "family."

Making New Memories

Though I was not feeling myself, Chris and I went on our annual Aruba vacation that we always took at the end of the summer with my sister and her family. I kept heeding the advice to keep things as normal as possible for me and Chris. Nothing is going to feel or be the same but maybe we could make some new memories.

While in Aruba, I visited my favorite jewelry store, Kay's Fine Jewelry (KFJ). Many years before, we purchased a ring as a replacement for my original engagement ring that was stolen during the break-in. My husband never offered to replace it and now I understand why. It was Lauren who said during our trip that mom had to have a new diamond ring. So, with her insistence, I got a gorgeous three-stone ring that I had always wanted and of course Lauren said, "Mommy three diamonds, for love, energy and power."

I was very friendly with the owner, Tesh, and asked what he might be able to do with my ring. I couldn't really wear it anymore but loved what Lauren said about the stones. He worked on a design and poured mimosas for me and Marion until he came up with a design for a beautiful, tiered pendant. As I took my ring off for the last time I cried and handed it over to him. He said he could have it ready the next day. It came out amazing and now reminds me of my girl every time I wear it. I would go back to KFJ to have more pieces made, each time to signify another milestone in my life. A girl has got to take care of herself and it was time I did just that.

More Dark Days

When Chris returned to school in the fall, I could not imagine the dark days that were ahead of me. I felt like everyone I loved left me – with no purpose for me to exist. My daughter was gone, my husband was gone and Chris was back at school. Nobody needed me anymore. I was having irrational thoughts and never imagined that I would have to utilize everything I had taught Lauren. Somehow, I had to find the strength within me to be stronger than I knew. I had to be the Warrior Princess and "suck it up" and continue on even though everything I loved and understood was taken away – not knowing even more adversity was still to come.

I told myself again and again this would be a time to really rediscover "me" and truly figure out who I am now while being fully accountable and aware of who I have been in the past as well as the present. I decided to look forward to creating a new version of me. One who knows true, unconditional love, joy and happiness. A life filled with trust, well-being, friends and maybe one day, true partnership. I knew this wouldn't happen overnight, but I *would* eventually get there.

The Great Pretender

For a long time to come, I would swirl in disbelief that the husband I knew could commit so many acts of betrayal and was actually gone. My heart had been shattered by the loss of Lauren and now my husband crushed what was left, trust destroyed, dreams obliterated. I'd shared my life for twenty-five years with a man I no longer recognized. Whoever he is now, he is not the man I once knew. He had become, and perhaps always was, *nothing* more than the "Great Pretender."

Even so, I was sad I would never grow old with the one person in my life who I shared a love with for so many years and who took the journey of Lauren with me. I was sad Chris would not have his father here to guide him and see the man he would grow to be after he graduated college. Finally, I was sad that someone I loved could hurt me so deeply and put me at risk for so many years without thought to what it would mean for us or our families. I could not understand how he could so easily discard us all.

Wusband

Some friends and family were shocked, others were not. One neighbor we were close with referred to him as my "wusband" which made me laugh and then sigh – because I knew he was right. Looking back from the time we met, I can see how it was *never* a healthy relationship or marriage. He truly had become *nothing* more than the man who *was* my husband.

They say everything happens for a reason and once again I had to trust that whatever was happening here could possibly have a silver lining. Perhaps my wusband and I were meant to be together to assist Lauren through her journey and that was all. I actually don't know what I would have done if I found out sooner. It would have crushed Lauren as well.

100% Responsible For Me

Now I had to find out what made me happy regardless of the choices made by others. I'm 100% responsible for me, I remembered from my time at Miraval. I always tried to make a beautiful life for us and for the family and have walked a path of integrity, light and service. I needed to consider that it perhaps was not in my best interest to hold onto a marriage where there were so many lies, so much betrayal and selfishness. He was a man who claimed one thing while doing another, would I want someone like that in my life?

For a long time, I felt like a victim and wondered how he could do "that" to me. I would soon come to understand how his actions made sense.

Sick and Tired

My wusband erased me from his narrative and limited our contact to email but would occasionally call to let me know of impending break-ups. It appeared he might be checking in to see if there was an opportunity with me, but I knew it was more about his fear of being alone. I did wonder each time if he had woken up from his past mistakes and perhaps wanted to make amends. Without fail, he would be back in his relationship in less than two weeks and back to no communication. His calls had a way of smacking me back into anger and sadness.

It all took a toll on me. My head literally spun, and I started having regular bouts of vertigo, back pain, ear pain and episodes of nausea. For the next two years, I would suffer from these on-and-off again symptoms. I even got an MRI to get to the root cause. It appeared to be the result of nothing more than stress and anxiety over the compounded losses I had experienced. The only thing that would help to alleviate the symptoms was rest. Many days I felt lost and wondered if I would ever snap out of this funk I was in. I had to find a way back, but how?

Getting Back to Happy

One morning, I watched a couple, Marc and Angel Chernoff, being interviewed on Megyn Kelly TODAY. They talked about a book they wrote called *Getting Back to Happy*. I listened intently as they shared their story and helpful insights from their book on how they overcame losses of their own. I ordered their book and found out about a workshop they were offering and decided to go. Maybe this would be the thing I needed to reboot my life.

While there, I volunteered to go on stage to get some live coaching. I shared my story of losing Lauren and my marriage and at a certain point said: "He shouldn't have done that to me." The leaders pointed out that while that may be true, there is another important question to ask.

"Isn't it also TRUE that a selfish person who thinks only of themselves would and could do such terrible things?" The answer to that is a resounding "YES!"

I learned by taking the time to ask, "Is this really true?" in any given situation, offered new insight into how I was framing the situation and whether it was helpful or even valid. I recognized that I was not the *victim* here and that a person's actions speak volumes about who *they* are and had nothing to do with me or anyone else. I was also reminded that hurting people hurt people. It all allowed me to put things in perspective.

This was the beginning of starting to feel good again and see things how they really were versus how I imagined them to be. It also felt good that so many people came up to me afterward to praise me for the courage to tell my story and how much it helped them.

Letting Go

After that, I became friendly with Marc and Angel, and from them I learned many things. I learned that letting go is an art; it has to do with stepping back and allowing things to happen. To trust that many things will take care of themselves and my needs will always be met. Believing this way would free me from the stress of trying to manage or control the situation. It gives me more time and energy to work on the things that truly matter – the things I actually can control, like my attitude and how I choose to respond.

This form of "letting go" is not giving up. It's about surrendering any obsessive attachments to specific people, outcomes and situations. It means I show up every day with the intention to be my best self, without expecting life to go a certain way. Having goals and dreams, taking purposeful action and building great relationships, while detaching from what I think every aspect of my life "must" look like in order to be "good enough" for me.

I'm here to live my best life and be the best version of me – that's exactly what I intend to do from here on out. That's what Lauren would want for me too. To continue to be kind, loving and caring and know that there are others out there who do the same. Though I had great loss, there is also great love. On that, I would not give up.

College Graduation

I really didn't want Christopher's graduation day to be the first time I saw my wusband since he left almost a year before and contacted him to ask if we could meet prior to the event. He told me he was breaking off his relationship "again" and agreed to come to New York early so we could talk. That meeting never happened. He texted me shortly before he was supposed to come to let me know he changed his mind, and it was no surprise to find that his relationship was back on.

My wusband went up to see Chris the day before the graduation. He took him skydiving and out to dinner. At the ceremony I sat with Marion and Chris' girlfriend, Kayla, who was a junior at SUNY Geneseo. Afterward we took pictures and Christopher's father left to catch a flight. The rest of us continued to celebrate the day and went to a party at the rugby house before going out to dinner at our favorite restaurant. I'm sure it was a bittersweet occasion for Chris.

Unconditional Love

I wanted Chris to have something to look forward to when he came home and decided to get him a puppy as part of his graduation present. Kayla searched online in the weeks prior and found a little black lab, a rescue puppy. We still had Jasper but he was about fourteen years old now and just about had enough energy to eat and sleep. It was important to me that Chris returned to a house filled with unconditional love and what better way to do that than with his very own puppy? I picked up the puppy on my way home from graduation so Chris could come home to find him waiting. (And he could help me train him over the summer!)

He was so excited and definitely brought such good energy back into the house. He named him Xander after his favorite Boston Red Sox player, who happens to be from Aruba! It was good to see Chris so happy again. There is truth to the saying that there is nothing better than a boy and his dog. He was everything Chris wanted in a dog, playful, fun and lots and lots of energy.

Time to Move On

It was time to enjoy the summer and a new puppy! Xander kept us both busy and filled our home with joy and puppy magic. Chris would soon begin his job search and I was looking forward to helping him get his new life started as well as my own.

Later that summer, I planned a trip to Montreal to see my friend, Ann, when I got a call from my wusband asking if we could meet. He said he needed to get away and was going to be spending some time in New York at his parents' house. It turned out he would be flying in while I was away but would still be in town when I got back. I agreed to meet him for lunch. This time he did show up and told me how he was once again in the middle of a breakup, with boxes already packed. He explained how he hasn't been himself since he left and feels numb all the time.

Then he said, "I'm moving to a new apartment – alone – and I wanted to see if we could have a different kind of relationship and thought maybe you could come and visit." *Whaaat the what?*, I thought to myself. Visit him after the way he treated me this past year? I didn't know exactly what he was thinking, but I had to let him know I no longer trusted anything he had to say and too much time and hurt had gone by for us to have a "relationship" of any kind or for me to come visit.

I was, however, always willing to talk and try to do some healing. At the end of lunch, it still felt there was so much left unsaid between us. After all we had gone through together, it always made me sad the way he ended things and how he chose to behave after he left. Two weeks later (as usual), he had a roommate back and communications ceased. To move on completely, I needed to finalize the divorce. It was time.

One-Two-Three Punch

Just as I was working on finalizing my divorce, my company of thirty-plus years announced that they were being acquired. There were rumors they would be laying off and selling many parts of the organization, including mine. This job was all I had left of my identity. It also provided financial security and benefits for me and Chris. What was I going to do now?

At first, this was almost too much to bear. Within a three-year span, I had lost my daughter, my marriage, and now my job might be coming to an end. How much can one person endure? I was brought to my knees again by this third unexpected blow and referred to what was happening in my life as the one-two-three punch – leaving me feeling beaten up, doubled over in pain, unable to breathe from repeated punches to the gut.

It would take months for the deal to settle and to find out for sure where things would end and what would happen when. It was another incredible time of more uncertainty and trepidation for me.

Blessings

I wouldn't find out until the very end of the acquisition that I was going to be kept on to assist with the transition of the training department for nine more months. This would mean more time to figure out what's next. It also promised a nice bonus for staying on in addition to a severance package. The timing of all of this was actually perfect and afforded me the opportunity to stay in my home that I loved, where I raised my children. I felt a sense of security I hadn't felt in a long time. Like God had given me what I needed to get back on track: time and resources to explore what I might want to do next.

Who knew that losing my job would turn out to be the biggest blessing and the easiest part of what I had to learn to let go of. Though, at the time, it was another moment that would rock my world when I was least prepared for it. I felt like I was stripped down to the core of all the things that defined me as a person.

Chris was still living at home, but he was working full-time and had plans to move out in a year. So, there would just be me. He got me a very special necklace for my birthday that year with the coordinates of our house and got me a beautiful card that said: "Home is wherever you are." He always seemed to know the right things to say and do, oh how I love that boy!

So many of my co-workers were in despair as well and I felt compelled to help in some way. I decided to offer weekly meditations in our corporate gym for as long as I was still an employee. I thought I would get a few people to show up but instead the gym was packed with people for each and every class. They thanked me so much for helping them with the breathing techniques I taught as well as the guided meditations and energy work I did at the end of each meditation. I used my Tibetan bowl to clear their chakras and provided them with essential oils. It felt good to be of service, using the skills I'd learned during my long journey of healing with my daughter.

I decided after my job ended that I would take some time off and go traveling. I didn't know where or with who, but that was my plan and it was going to be fabulous. The other thing I knew for sure was that I was going to use the time to finally write the book I always wanted to about Lauren's life.

Magic Whiteboard

I made a list on the whiteboard in my home office to include these and other things I wanted to accomplish in order to start my new life. I listed all the months of the year and next to it put what I hoped to complete. It included taking care of myself, expanding my network, buying a new car (one that I wanted), finding a new job, finalizing the divorce and, of course, taking a "fabu" trip and starting to write this book.

A year later, I looked back and realized everything on the whiteboard not only happened, but happened the exact month I imagined. I call it my "magic whiteboard." It's all part of the art of manifestation. It's important to set goals and be clear on your intentions and then take steps towards making them happen. I have always done vision boards around the New Year but this is the first time I laid it out on a white board and had every single thing happen!

Self-Care

First and foremost, it was time to start taking good care of myself. Stress causes a lot of problems, so I rested when I needed to rest. I joined a gym near my house that offered spin, yoga and meditation classes. I started a regular care program of getting facials and massages as well. I attended grief counseling at my church and later became a grief counselor myself.

I have journaled my whole life and continued to do so during all of this time. It brought clarity to how I was feeling, and I could also see my progress and growth from years past. Not only was journaling good for my soul, but when it came to writing this book, I had accurate accounts of everything that happened. It's amazing how much you forget after time goes by. I have come to find that writing can be an absolute cathartic experience.

Too Soon to Write?

I saw there was a course being offered at my library on "Writing Your Life Story" and decided to take it. That got my creative juices flowing. As I wrote, though, I had lots of emotions come up. I spoke to the instructor about it when I inquired about her book coaching and editing services. She told me that writing a book is much like the grieving process. It's never too late but sometimes it's too soon. She suggested I wait a bit and said, "when the story is ready, the pen will flow." A few months later I was in contact with her again and that's when the time felt right!

Fabulous Vacation

The trip came about when my niece Jessica, asked me if I wanted to go to the South Pacific with her. Her roommate was supposed to go but had to back out. The timing coincided with my job ending and seemed like it was meant to be. Everything seemed to be falling into place better than if I had planned it myself.

Just before I left, I found out my divorce was final. It was the day before the fourth of July and gave me a sense of freedom to go out on this adventure now, free and ready to discover what sparks joy for me. We spent a month traveling through Fiji, New Zealand, and Australia. I especially loved Australia where I went diving in the Great Barrier Reef, ate dinner and saw Madam Butterfly in the

Sydney Opera House, went to Bondi Beach and the Royal Botanical Garden and so much more. It was the trip of a lifetime and truly fabulous!

Synchronicity

When I got back from the South Pacific, I had a week before I was leaving to go on the annual trip to Aruba. I saw a job online that looked perfect for me and decided to apply. To my surprise, they called me immediately and asked how soon I could interview. When I told them I was leaving for vacation the following week, they set up a meeting for the very next day. The phone screen went well and when I returned, I finished the cycle of interviews and was offered the position.

I had not really intended to start work until the following year so I could take time off to relax, finish healing and work on my writing, but it was an opportunity I could not turn down. I would be working from home as a senior program manager for one of the top four companies in the world. I was really excited!

Life 2.0

I love my new job! I get to work with a great team for a great company doing great things. I mostly work from home with light travel, which couldn't be more perfect. I'm comfortably able to stay in my house until I feel I'm ready to leave. Life these days is completely on my terms.

I would have never imagined any of these things happening, not the bad or the good things that awaited me. It was inconceivable to me that Lauren one day would not be with me and that I would have to apply all the things I taught her to myself when facing my own dark times. It was incomprehensible that my wusband could betray me for years and never let on until he was good and ready to go. It was unimaginable that I would lose my job at a company I had worked at for over thirty years. It was a triple play of the most unbearable things anyone would ever have to endure.

Not Where I Used to Be

Getting back to happy for me has been a long, slow climb. Kind of like climbing Mt. Kilimanjaro, Pole, pole (Slowly, slowly). Now that I think about it, I don't think you actually get or find "happy." I think you just take steps that move you in the direction you want to head and let happiness and joy find you. I'm not completely there yet, but I definitely have more and more "happy" moments. I guess you could say I'm not where I want to be, but I'm sure not where I used to be.

Forgiveness

I've read a lot about forgiveness and know it takes a long time to get there, but the most important thing I learned is that to forgive is for oneself and does not let the other person off the hook. In all the years that have gone by since my wusband left, he never once asked me to forgive him. I started with forgiving myself and in doing so, I was able to release the pain and anger of the past and found a way to work through the unimaginable for a second time around.

Labor of Love

Through writing this book, Lauren has taken me on yet another journey. What I've come to realize is that though Lauren was the one who was blind, I was the one who could not see. Now I'm awake with eyes wide open, I can clearly see all the signposts that I missed while I was busy "doing" instead of "being." I have found through all of this that I truly am stronger than I know – I think we all are. Putting these words down has now also let me put the story down. What I take from here is what I've had all along – her love.

CHAPTER

Twenty Three

Reflections Of Lauren

Lauren touched the lives of so many and somehow seems to have transcended death through her light, beauty and love. I could not tell you her story without telling you part of mine, but I'd like to bring the focus back to Lauren and share the light she was in this world and continues to be, the beauty she brought by the positive and colorful way she lived her life and the love she shared so freely and unconditionally.

I couldn't think of a better way to do this than by sharing words from her best friend, Lulu. In this chapter, Lulu shares her reflections on what life was like growing up with Lauren and what that friendship has meant to her. I think it's a perfect example of the impact Lauren has had on others and how her spirit lives on each and every day and the impact she has had in this world.

Point of Power

"I remember meeting Lauren at a classmate's birthday party when we were in fourth grade. At the party, there was one of those big blow-up slides in front of the house. I was standing behind Lauren waiting for my turn on the slide and said, "Hi Lauren – I'm in Mrs. J's class with you." It stuck out to me that Lauren always dressed really nice in great matching outfits and pocketbooks. This day was no different and Lauren had on cuffed blue jeans with white Keds sneakers and wore a black sweater that had a puffy poodle on it with a heart around it. She topped it off with a cross over shoulder bag that had her gum and lip gloss in it.

Lauren had the best sense of humor and I remember how we would take walks to the library and we'd put on accents or pretend to be a celebrity. She especially liked speaking with an English accent or valley girl. I would pretend to be someone famous and Lauren would go along with it like she was being fooled. It was so much fun, and we laughed as others looked strangely at us.

I remember how goofy Lauren was – in the best way – and how fun she was to be with.

She always amazed me with her positive disposition, even while losing her vision. She was always ready and proud to show others what she could do in Braille when other students were curious. Lauren was more than happy when I asked her for the first time if she could read a book to me in Braille: "Of course," Lauren said. I was so impressed by her and her ability to adapt and keep her positivity.

You could always count on more laughs when Lauren was in the classroom. She had a lot of times where she had to pulled out of class for all her therapies and activities due to her low vision, but whenever she was there the whole class was excited about it. Lauren had a contagious positivity, and her perspective was so pure because she didn't have any preconceived notions about what someone looked like. She was super genuine all the time.

Even though Lauren was legally blind and walked with a cane, we would talk about what it would be like to drive a car when we turned sixteen and how exciting that would be. That is how optimistic she was! It didn't matter what her abilities were, whether she could see or not, she was just as much appreciative of all the things around her as everyone else, which I thought was pretty fantastic. I was always so impressed that nothing seemed to phase Lauren at all – not when she needed to start using a cane and not when she had to learn Braille. It was just a part of who she was and she was ok with all of it. Not being able to see almost seemed like a 'point of power' for her.

Maybe this is how she was able to connect with people on a deeper level because she didn't have that surface level opinion that we all have in our lives which prevents us from being able to really see each other. She turned something that a lot of people would just sink into and be sad about or feel like they need pity for and deprived of the world around them – but she was able to connect with everyone around her as well as her surroundings in order to be able to navigate the world with the sight and vision she had. I think it made her attuned and allowed her to operate on a different wavelength and everyone around her could feel that.

277

She saw everyone's potential for beauty and perfection. Everyone had an equal opportunity with Lauren, and she offered them the opportunity to embrace her view of the world and greatness. She always approached everyone in the exact same way, which was arms and heart wide open, ready to give and learn about you from the very first second. She did this by asking a zillion questions about your life. When you answered her questions, all she would do is wish greatness upon you. It didn't matter what your answers were.

She would always tell me how beautiful I was and how I was going to find a boyfriend one day who loved me more than anything. And she would always have a list of adjectives to describe the life she wished for you: amazing, magnificent, incredible and you would be like, 'when is it going to end?' – but it was so precious and genuine. That was her vision of how great everyone was and level of respect and love everyone deserved. She gave that to everyone, no matter who you were, it was up to you to accept her offer or not.

She taught me how to do the same and live HPH. By that, I mean I live by kind of being blind to people at first and approach someone with that same full and open heart that Lauren did. I try not to ever think ill of someone before I have got the chance to talk with them. Even after I talk with them and maybe don't agree with them, I realize they still deserve all the goodness life has to offer and maybe they are just not the friend or person for me.

There have been many times I have applied her philosophies of life where I don't think I would have gotten through as easily without them. When my sister got cancer, I relied on having faith in the best outcome possible and that is a quality Lauren had. She had a faith-filled optimism towards everything. She was devoted to

278

spreading light in the world and making people feel better and she made herself feel better at the same time. I think that's what drove her for so long. It was the impact she made on people and continues to make even after she passed. When my sister, Sophie, was going through her chemo, I was able to look at it as an opportunity to bond and strengthen ourselves and persevere versus having pity or thinking the worst.

Lauren won many battles and in my eyes it was because of her faith and positivity. The fact that she could coin a phrase, "Happy, Positive and Healthy" during a time filled with so many challenges is nothing less than incredible. The first time I heard this phrase was in middle school after she got back to school from her six-month hospitalization.

She left shortly after sixth grade started and came back in eighth grade. I remember it being so hard for her that year, but she always did her best. She was still the same goofy Lauren telling her jokes and wanting to make everyone laugh. She also brought something with her to give out every day whether it was a Werther candy, a bracelet or just a hug. On the day of our eighth-grade graduation, we wore our hair the same way, in a pony off to the side. She looked beautiful in a long purple dress with sequins on top – again always so fashionable!

When it was decided Lauren would be going to a different high school, I would still go over to see her and spend time when I could. I would bring my guitar and sing songs with her and she always liked to hear me play. We would talk like valley girls and Lauren would include phrases like "Totally", "Whatever" and "Oh My God" and use the word "Like" as much as possible. We would laugh like we did back in sixth grade.

For her sweet sixteen, I got her a necklace that said HPH on it because that is always what Lauren embodied to me. I didn't know at the time what her diagnosis was and how little time I would have left with my best friend. Less than a year later, she passed.

As heartbroken as I was to lose Lauren, she taught me so much and has become such a blessing and literally helps me through every situation in my life. It's hard but it's also so so so beautiful and that's what I try to think of when I think of Lauren — that I'm so lucky to have met someone who has impacted me so much. She is love and brought pure genuine light and joy into this world. If I am ever having a bad day, I think of Lauren and her philosophies on life and they really do guide me through. Lauren dealt with so much and she was astronomically more positive than I ever am at any given point in time. I can now embody that. After I think about and make myself aware, I can always push through.

There was a time during my senior year in college when I was going through a breakup with my boyfriend. I was so anxious and crying all the time. I felt half livid, half super-depressed and so just not wanting to get out of bed in the morning and not wanting to deal with the imminent failure of my relationship. I was feeling so sorry for myself and not being kind to myself in my head and wallowing in my despair. I would think about how hopeless I felt in that moment and then I would curl over and see the HPH tattoo I have on my left forearm — strategically placed on the inner arm so it falls by my heart — and think about Lauren. Or I would go for a drive and pick up my keys that have her bracelet with stars, butterflies and hearts and I would hold them in my hand for an extra second longer and realize that everything in this moment, I'm able to overcome and I have to put on a brave face.

When I raise my arm up, those three little letters, HPH, are next to my head and I can almost hear Lauren whispering to me for a little bit. It's such a part of me that I wanted it physically on my body for the rest of my life. Curious people ask me about it. At first, they think it's someone's initials but I tell them HPH stands for Happy, Positive and Healthy and they think that's cute, but they don't really understand the depth of it. Then I go on to tell them all about Lauren and how she fully lost her vision by age eleven and what a tough life she had and then I go on to tell them she is the most inspirational person I ever met in my life. It somehow has a profound effect on them.

I would add that Lauren didn't see herself as sick or a girl with a brain tumor or anything else. She self-diagnosed herself as HPH – Happy, Positive and Healthy and that's exactly what she lived by ALL the time. That's exactly what she spread by handing out bracelets filled with love, energy and power. People always cry when I tell them her story. They say I'm sorry – and I tell them not to be. She lived a really beautiful life. She impacted me and now she just impacted you and you get to take her wherever you go. That was her offering to people, in the physical at least, and now I carry her love with me everywhere I go.

I can see the impact it has on them by their smile and their eyes are gleaming from this tiny little perspective that has the potential to change their life. Lauren's love is exponentially growing around us from this. I know people from high school and see them on social media and see them still wearing Lauren's bracelets all these years later. Lauren is never far from me and all those she has touched.

I was so honored that I was asked to sing at Lauren's funeral mass. It's not the first time I sang "Somewhere Over the Rainbow/ What a Beautiful World" at a funeral, but it would be the most difficult. That song is so touching and has a similar message to what Lauren was all about – that there is beauty in everything and to spread that happiness and beauty – and she just did that so perfectly. I can't hear or play that song without a tear rolling down my face.

Signs of Lauren are everywhere. Like the time shortly after I started college in SUNY New Paltz. I was going through a really tough time – overwhelmed with life away from home and all the school work. I looked up at the sky and saw a smiley face and immediately thought of Lauren. I continued to look around for more hints of her and couldn't believe it but I could clearly see the letters: H P H in the sky. It served as a reminder to always "look up" and know her love is never far and Lauren's light is all around us.

CHAPTER

Twenty Four

Take A Chance

There are moments in life, if we are lucky, when we are presented with what can be considered a "once-in-a-lifetime opportunity" to do or see something incredible. Life with Lauren presented me with many of those opportunities and for that I will be forever grateful. Sometimes it involves taking a chance to go out of our comfort zone, trying something new or making ourselves vulnerable.

For me, writing this book is one of those times. Sharing details of my life with Lauren and reliving the pain of losing her and the challenges and shocks that followed was a chance I took in hopes this could help even one person who may be going through something similar.

Chance the Rapper

The summer after Lauren passed, Chris found out Chance the Rapper was going to be playing in Toronto, Canada. He not only loved Chance's music but also loved what a good person he was. Chance focused on helping people in his hometown of Chicago by donating to many local causes and was just a "good dude" as Christopher put it.

It was a four-hour ride from his college and none of his friends wanted to go, but he wasn't going to let that stop him from a chance to see his favorite artist. He decided to go and pay the extra money to get a VIP ticket, which included a meet and greet and early entry to the standing-room only concert.

Chris made the drive in our mini-van (the only car we would let him drive up at school) and arrived early. He then waited on line for three hours for his two minutes with Chance. When he finally met him, he said, "Hey, I just want to say I love your music and I really appreciate everything you're doing." Then he added, "I have also been through a pretty tough time this past year." He explained, "I recently lost my sister and your music has been really uplifting to me and has helped me get through it."

Chance then said, "Ah, man – I'm really sorry to hear that, and I'm glad I was able to be an inspiration to you."

Chris took the opportunity to share how Lauren made her special bracelets and told him how she put love, energy and power in every bead and said to Chance, "I'd appreciate you having one," and handed him a bracelet. He really didn't expect him to do anything with it and thought Chance would just put it aside with all the other items he received from his fans and didn't really give it any more thought.

Once In a Lifetime Moment

Since Chris arrived so early, he got one of the best spots in the house and got to stand right up against the stage. During the opening act, Chance came out to join the warm-up performer and Chris noticed he still had Lauren's bracelet on and was moved to tears. He thought, "Holy $#!%" this guy cares so much and understood how important this was to me, someone he didn't know, someone from a totally different background – how cool is that – that he was wearing it."

Chance went off stage and when he came back on for his solo performance, Chris was shocked that he still had the bracelet on. Then Chance looked over and saw Chris and as they exchanged glances, Chance told the audience this next song is for everyone out there who has ever gone through a tough time and raised the arm up that he was wearing Lauren's bracelet on. He then looked at Chris and smiled and shook his head as if to say:

"Yeah man, I get that we all go through tough times," and acknowledged him in a way that was so incredibly special.

Her Love Continues to Spread

Chris will never forget the experience he had at that concert. He took a chance, going alone, and what followed was certainly one of the once-in-a-lifetime moments when he got to see his sister's love, energy and power in action.

Chance exhibited it by choosing to wear Lauren's bracelet and held up his wrist for all to see – with words and reverberation of love, energy and power among the audience – who did not know about the bracelet, but who did know what Chance was conveying. He was speaking love, he was showing power and unity, and the whole event was energy.

This brought Lauren's philosophy to life in that very moment. Through Chris' life and his experiences – her love continues – serendipity at its best.

CHAPTER

Twenty Five

Love, Energy And Power

Christopher and Lauren are the two greatest loves in my life. Music is another shared love that was an important part of our lives. We danced to it, sang to it and cried from it. Some songs told a story while others just had a great beat. Lauren loved to listen to all kinds of music from country to pop and loved to sing to her favorite songs. During her hospital stay we found out about an organization called "Songs of Love" and she even had a custom song written about her and was recorded in her favorite genre, country. She was thrilled and would play it over and over. Music always had a special way to lift us up and makes us feel good.

Hand of God

Christopher was greatly impacted by music and the artists he admires. He loved a song by Jon Bellion (a Long Island artist) called "Hand of God" which is the outro song on the album "The Human Condition." The words in that song expressed things he could not. He made a comparison to life being just like this song, which incorporates lyrics from all the other songs on the album and builds and builds with incredible brass and strings and gospel like emotion. It represents to Chris how life is a culmination of all our past experiences and how many things are not in our control and how you need to take the positives out of it all and be the best version of yourself – the way Lauren did!

He asked his girlfriend, Kayla, to design a tattoo that beautifully represents the combination of what this song meant and the wisdom his sister imparted on him. Words of reference are:

"I am just a man, I am just a man, who lusts, gives, tries, sometimes I lose my way.

Tears at a funeral, tears at a funeral, I might break.

Angry at all the things, angry at all the things, I can't change.

When you're lost in the universe, lost in the universe, Don't lose faith!

My mother says, "Your whole life is in the hands of God."

The tattoo is a hand with an open palm holding a star, butterfly and heart with lowercase letters "hph" underneath it. He has the tattoo over his heart. It is symbolic of the love for his sister and the message she shared. I love that tattoo and what it represents so much. Kayla had a picture made of it on pink canvas and gave it to me to for Christmas.

Tattoo Brigade

My sister, Marion, and her three daughters, Jessica, Julianne and Kelcie also got special tattoos in honor of Lauren. Each one specially designed and placed to remind them of their cousin and her philosophy. For example, Jessie had an LC with angel wings tattooed on her left hand to have Lauren with her for big life events – that would be the hand she wears a wedding ring on and the arm she would hold a baby with. Julianne put a cross on her wrist to remind her to always have faith and know that Lauren is with God. Kelcie put the symbols of love, energy and power on her right foot to signify that she would always be walking forward with Lauren. Even my next-door neighbor Keith, who we only knew for little over a year at the time, was so touched and got a big colorful butterfly tattoo with the initial L.C. on his arm.

They tried to convince me to get a tattoo for her too, but that's just not me. I didn't want or need a tattoo on my body to remind me of the love I carry with me each and every moment of every day. She has left an impression deeper than any tattoo could ever leave behind.

Live HPH

There are so many more stories from Lauren's friends, family members, neighbors and even total strangers where she has had a similar impact, but it is just too much to share here in the book. This story of Lauren's Vision stands to represent how she touched so many people in her short but impactful lifetime. Those lives who have been touched by this angel will never be the same, especially mine.

In this world, there is so much loss and pain – but at the same time there is so much joy and love. It's inevitable to experience all these things at some point. You can see the glass as half-empty or half-full. I never let Lauren see the glass as half-empty for one second. In turn, she embodied a light that shined so brightly people could feel it in her presence. Many of us face this same decision every day when we wake up and can choose, like I did, to get out of our bed (or not).

So, I will leave you with this to think about...

What story do you tell yourself?

Which wolf will you feed?

What thoughts will you allow yourself to continue to think, be, do and have?

I choose to continue Lauren's Vision of being a hug collector, laughing often, living HPH and spreading her message of LOVE, ENERGY and POWER.

I hope you do the same.

Lauren's HPH Fund / How To Get A Bracelet

All proceeds from this book are being donated to the Lauren Cummins HPH Fund, a Fidelity Giving Account, established in March 2020. Every year, in honor of Lauren's birthday, a portion of this account will be donated to a charity so that the giving can go on forever, just like her love. Anyone who makes a donation to Lauren's fund is eligible to receive a bracelet.

For more information on Lauren's fund or how to get a bracelet, visit www.laurensvision.com.

Signing off...

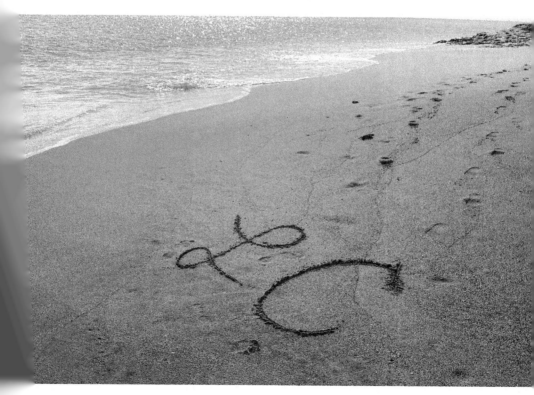

AFTERWORD

I could have never imagined when I started writing that I would be completing this book about love, loss and learning to live again during a pandemic when so many people would be experiencing the same. Never has there been a time in our history where there has been so much global fear, uncertainty and doubt about what the future holds.

This book has been a labor of love and there were three things I hoped to accomplish. First and foremost, I wanted to share the beauty and joy of Lauren and the amazing, positive life she lived despite all the challenges she faced. It was difficult to pick only some of the stories of how she inspired others around her with her amazing philosophy of living HPH. There were so many others she touched, those she knew and those who only heard stories of her – both while she lived and after she died. This child was a true light and beamed with happiness. I'd like to think I had a small part of infusing her with that but mostly that was who she was at her core. It is without doubt this child completed her soul's purpose and ready to make her journey home. She made that clear to me as we went on her last walk as she softly said the last words we would ever hear her say: "I want to go home now."

Second, it's my hope to inspire and uplift anyone who has had obstacles to overcome from loss of any kind, confronted unexpected adversities, or experienced a major life change. While the loss of a child or any loved one is devastating, I learned the love you shared stays with you always. I've also come to learn that the loss of a

293

marriage or even a job, while at a different level, is still hard, and you have to find a way to begin again. The support you get from your faith, family and friends is immeasurable. So whether you are a mother, father, sister, brother, any other family member, caretaker, nurse, doctor, therapist, teacher, neighbor or friend of a loved one who is facing any one of these challenges, I hope this has in some way helped you see what the family and individual might be going through. We all need to be treated as a whole person, with love and kindness and know we are more alike than different.

Last, I wanted to share the spiritual journey I took and how much comfort faith brought to both me and Lauren as difficulties increased. I hope others will not judge the unorthodox things I pursued and tried until they have walked a mile in my shoes. It was not my intention to change anyone's thoughts or beliefs about Spirit but rather to share my journey as someone who struggled with her own relationship with God and faith. I was trying to understand what it means to have faith and struggling to make sense of things that seemed senseless to me. I wanted to share how my eyes opened to the unseen world and the new relationship I cultivated with God and spirit. It was a comfort for me to know that I am never alone during times when I felt so isolated. I always knew no matter what happened, I had a choice about how I could respond. I never blamed God for anything that happened. I believe God uses all things for good and it was up to me to find the silver lining and put my best foot forward regardless of the circumstances. I have found that as long as I keep walking in the direction I want to head, I will ultimately get there. As Lauren's doctor always said, you never know what's around the corner. I always chose to focus on the positive in my life

294

and what it could be and stopped at nothing until I got there. Lauren lived her best life because of it. I now try to do the same.

If I have touched your life in any way by sharing these experiences, then I have accomplished what I set out to do. This book is the legacy I leave on my daughter's behalf and I hope you feel inspired, uplifted and know beyond a shadow of a doubt that we are all stronger than we know and here to live life the way Lauren Visioned it, Happy, Positive and Healthy with Love, Energy and Power!

Never give up hope, never give up on love and always be good and kind to yourself and others!

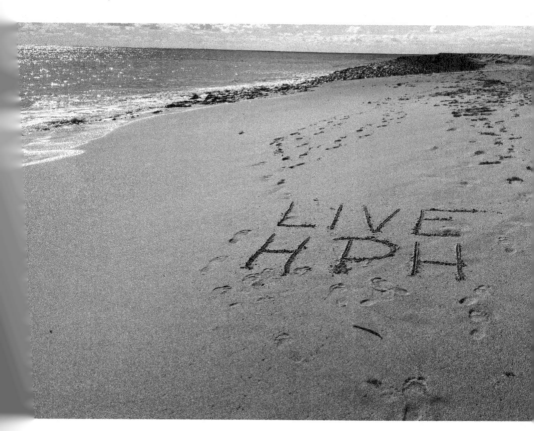

ACKNOWLEDGEMENTS

To my two beautiful children, Christopher and Lauren. You are the sunshine in my life and my reason to smile. You both have taught me about what it is to give and receive love unconditionally and how effortless that can be. It's been my honor and privilege to be your mother and assist you on your journey here and you, in turn, have assisted me on mine. The love from you, as well as from our family and friends, along with my faith has seen me through the best and worst of times. I would not have been able to keep going, growing and loving without all of it.

Chris, you have grown into the amazing man I always knew you would be. You have wisdom, strength and compassion beyond your years. I am so proud of you, the choices you have made and the man you have become.

Lauren, you will forever be my beautiful, amazing, loving, sweet baby girl. You touched my life in a way that is beyond words. You taught me how precious life is and to live HPH. I promise to spread your message of love, energy and power. I love and miss you every day.

To my family, thank you all for your love and support. You have been there for me, Lauren and Chris through it all and I'm so grateful for each and every one of you. I'd like to thank my mom, Linda and my late father, Ed Kalten for their love and for helping to shape me into the person I am today. My sisters and brothers are all a source of strength to me, thank you to Marion, her husband Jeff, Annalise, Eddie, David and Cathy. Special thanks to my nieces and nephews, Jessica, Michael, Julianne, Kelcie and Brayden, who were like siblings to Lauren and cushioned her with love.

To the Cummins, Breslin's and Lang's, who I will always consider my family, thank you for the love you have shown throughout the years and all the support you gave to our family.

To Maritza Febo and Lisa O'Connell, thank you for your friendship and being my BFFs. I don't know where I would be without either of you. Maritza, you are my spiritual rock and advisor and provide me the comfort of your shoulder to cry on whenever it's needed. Lisa, you are the voice of reason in all matters and my expert troubleshooter and financial buddy. Thank you both for being the best friends a girl could have!

To all my girls, Carly, Amanda, Brittnay, Toni, Emily, Dani, Lauren B, Jessie (my niece who needs to be included here too) and the countless other aides who helped me love and care for Lauren. Your friendship, laughter and love meant the world to me and to Lauren.

To Trish and Dan Daly, John (fancy pants) D'Arcy, Carder Kelly and Bryan Kudlek, thank you for sharing your love with my girl and making her feel special. She loved you all!

To Judy Grant and Bill Bezmen, thank you for spiritual guidance, workshops and friendship through the years. You are both a true blessing.

To everyone that was part of my beta-reader program, thank you for your invaluable feedback.

Special thanks to Kayla Kucerak (now Christopher's fiancée) who by reading the beta version not only provided invaluable feedback but also took a very special journey of Lauren and brought us ever closer together. I love you and so glad you are a part of our family!

To my writing coach and editor, Diane Riis of Earth and Soul Publishing, thank you for your assistance to map out the first rough draft of this book. Your encouragement to write the story that needed to be told and then wait for as long as it took to decide on the parts that I truly wanted to share was a very healing process. Your amazing ability to remix words allowed me to articulate what I was feeling far better than I ever could have without your expert guidance.

To Ann Papayoti, my good friend, author, life coach, fitness enthusiast and person extraordinaire – thank you for all your love, support and encouragement to get the final draft finished and published. I'm honored you wrote the foreword and look forward to other projects.

To all of Lauren's friends, especially the Miller Place graduating class of 2016, for your love and friendship. There are too many of you to mention but you all rock!

To the Miller Place School District faculty and staff and the Samoset special education team who supported Lauren through it all and made sure she had everything she needed. Thank you, thank you, thank you!

To the many doctors, nurses, residents, social workers, counselors, child life therapists, volunteers and all the other medical professionals, caregivers and staff who provided care for Lauren, thank you for all you do for your patients and their families. Especially the staff at Stonybrook University Hospital (SBUH) and New York University Hospital (NYUH), what you do on a daily basis is nothing less than incredible.

To the staff and volunteers at Make-A-Wish of Long Island, Give Kids the World, Ronald McDonald House, Friends of Karen and the Sunshine Foundation, thank you for the care and support you provide to families like ours. You made our days a little easier and a bit brighter. You touch many hearts with your kindness and generosity and can't thank you enough.

To Tesh Chugani, thank you for your love, support and friendship throughout the years and during the writing of this book. Thank you, too, for making me and Lauren shine with your beautiful jewelry.

To Marc and Angel Chernoff for their wisdom and assistance on helping me find my way back to happy and for their advanced book praise. You truly help others redefine what's possible.

To Adrianne Yule who graciously gave her time to provide feedback while doing the copy editing of the final version of this book, thank you so much.

There have been many people that have since come into my life and proven you never know what lies around the corner. To the scientist I sat next to on a plane, who told me about a new treatment that provides five precious years for GBM patients, thanks for validating to never lose hope. To the new and special friends I have made who have shown me how to fun again and spark joy in my life, thank you. For those yet to come, I can't wait to meet you!

Each and every one of you are the real heroes in my life and have helped me in ways that are immeasurable through all the incredible loss and adversity. You have helped me to put the pain of the past down, to grow, to love and continue to live HPH. For that and so much more I thank you all.

ABOUT THE AUTHOR

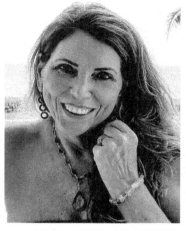

E. Lisa Cummins, PMP, CSPO is an IT professional. She holds a BS in business, has worked in the corporate world for over thirty-five years, and is a board member for PMI-LIC. She volunteers for charitable organizations, believes in holistic approaches to well-being and holds multiple certifications in alternative approaches to healing.

Lisa wants to share her late daughter's unconditional love and light with the world. She hopes to remind people that when we lose our loved ones, we don't lose their love. By sharing the amazing journey she took with Lauren, she hopes to offer others strength in their darkest times, and to help others on their own love and loss voyages.

She currently resides in Long Island, New York with her puppy Forest who'll go on to be a Guide Dog.